FRANK ZANE
MIND, BODY, SPIRIT

FRANK ZANE
MIND, BODY, SPIRIT

by Frank Zane, M.A.
3 times Mr. Olympia

drawings by Christine Zane, M.A., M.S.

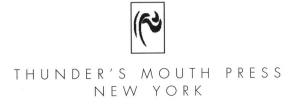

THUNDER'S MOUTH PRESS
NEW YORK

Published by
Thunder's Mouth Press
632 Broadway, Seventh Floor
New York NY 10012

Library of Congress Cataloging-in-Publication Data
Zane, Frank.
     Frank Zane mind, body, spirit / by Frank Zane ; drawings by Christine Zane.
        p.   cm.
     ISBN 1056025-112-3 (pbk.)
     1. Physical fitness. 2. Bodybuilding. 3. Weight training.
   4. Zane, Frank. I. Title.
GV481.Z356 1997
613.7'1—dc21   97-16514
                                                                                                      CIP

Dedicated to my mother, Laura G. Zane (1915-1996)
who built my body

INTRODUCTION

by Joe Weider

editor in chief, *Muscle & Fitness, Flex*

Knowing Frank Zane for over three decades, I have watched him develop into one of the greatest bodybuilders of all time. Being the leanest bodybuilder ever to win all the top titles, Mr. America, Mr. Universe, Mr. World, and Mr. Olympia, his 185 pound physique gave new meaning to the concepts of muscular balance, definition, symmetry, and proportion. He has the rare distinction of winning over Arnold Schwarzenegger in the 1968 Mr. Universe, mainly because Frank's attention to developing the fine details of all the muscles of the body, even the little ones.

Frank has been a contributing writer to *Muscle & Fitness* magazine since 1963, and in that time not only has he won the major bodybuilding competitions, he has also taught high school mathematics for 13 years (Frank tutored Arnold in college algebra in the early 1970's), earned a master's degree in psychology, received a California Life Teaching Credential, patented the Leg Blaster™ exerciser, teaches bodybuilding at his Palm Springs Zane Experience Seminars, and has published four successful books.

In *Frank Zane Mind, Body, Spirit*, his fifth book, Zane presents a pioneering blend of workout information and personal growth psychology. It is so many things in one book—hundreds of workout, aerobic training, nutrition, psychology, dreams, unique meditation techniques, motivational and inspirational advice from Frank's meticulously kept diaries dating back to the beginning of his 40 year bodybuilding career—all this is distilled into a 365 day-by-day progressive format anyone can use as an instructional guide to self-improvement. It is difficult to describe *Frank Zane Mind, Body, Spirit* in a single sentence except to say that it takes bodybuilding to new heights.

Frank Zane Mind, Body, Spirit's most important emphasis is the interaction of mind, body, and spirit. It is more than you'd expect even from someone such as Zane, who has brought mental training into bodybuilding like no one else has. Meditation, self-hypnosis, visualization, affirmations, dichotic and beat frequency audio tapes—all of this and more have taken him into the spiritual foundations of the human body, as he re-imagines the gym as both a physical excercise center as well as a place for personal transformation.

Frank Zane Mind, Body, Spirit expresses the beauty of the inner form or higher self, as well as the outer form and how to build it. Although it is packed full of sophisticated training information, at its deepest levels Frank's diaries are inspirational texts to be read for guidance and self-unfoldment both in bodybuilding practice and in personal life outside the gym. It is essential reading for beginners, as well as advanced bodybuilders of all ages.

Joe Weider

Frank Zane Mind, Body, Spirit is an organized and detailed training plan for men and women based on my 40-year training career. These diaries can guide you through each day of your training year—and for the rest of your life—as well as serve as a source of inspiration for workouts, nutrition, deep relaxation, entrainment by sound and light, meditation, motivation, dreams, mental discipline, and reduction of stress. Reading this book will help you understand that building muscle shape and definition demand that you follow the program closely in good form using whatever weights you can. You can refer to the exercise index in the back of the book or my book Fabulously Fit Forever for more information on the specific exercises mentioned throughout the book.

The Winter plan includes workouts about three times a week. For the Spring, the training regime becomes three days out of six. In Summer, the workouts increase to three days out of five. And at the beginning of the Fall, the frequency of training advances to three days out of four. With this system you will define your physique, just as nature defines four seasons:

Winter's a season with maintenance as its theme.
Spring time means growing depicted by the color green.
Summer's intensity is glowing lava red hot.
Autumn is maturity, harvest, ripeness, not rot.

Out of shape? Start January 1 and take it one day at a time doing the program for the day. Some days are workouts while on rest days I give you something to think about relating to the process of growth. If you have been training regularly you can begin in March and continue from there as the program gradually intensifies into Summer and leads to reaching your peak in early Autumn. Then a gradual downshifting into Winter along with a sense of appreciation of your progress.

I give the weights that I have personally used in these workouts. These are my poundages, not necessarily yours, so feel free to use whatever weights you are capable of handling in good form. The best way to do weight training is to use lighter weights at first with slow negatives (that is, return the weight to starting position slowly) using a rhythmic movement. You will extract the most benefit from lighter weights and your strength will grow. As a result you will gradually be able to handle heavier poundages in good form. Do this if you want your muscles to grow; if not, stay with lighter weights and cut down on the amount of rest you take between sets.

This is your diary so please write in all the spaces. And don't be afraid to write down the first things that come to mind. These are the most intuitive, insightful, and creative.

NOTE

A bracket or parentheses in front of two exercises means this a "super-set", that is a set the second exercise is done immediately after a set of the first exercise with any rest in between. Then the sequence is repeated.

A bracket in front of three exercises indicates a "tri-set", that is one set of each of three exercises is done with no rest between sets.

Example:

Super Set

{
reverse curl
   2 sets of 10 reps
wrist curl
   2 sets of 15 reps

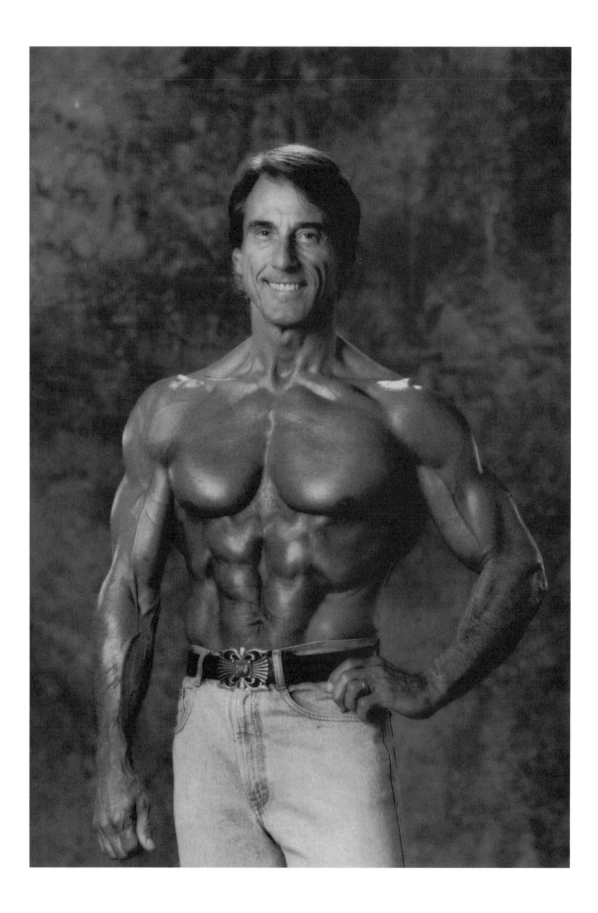

WINTER DIARY

40 years of my life's typical days
lay emblazened in these pages.

Lives of men and women might be delineated thus:
1. creation or coming into being
2. building the place for living
3. learning how to best live in the building
These three facts describe the whole life process.
At first we may wander about
wondering what and where is best for us.
Before long we find our spot
and begin construction with materials found
in the ground: sand, stone, ores, trees, clay
we build this house of us
in our own unique way
following the rules of carpentry.
The blueprint comes first and with this plan in mind
I lay my foundation in long straight lines
cementing cinder block upon block
balanced level construction
now there's no time for talk
and soon my walls are erected by noon.
My focus is keen
my building is begun
and everyone has seen
the building process is fun.

HERE ARE THE HIGHLIGHTS OF MY DAYS:

I'm just like you. I find it necessary to look for ways to motivate myself to train. The search has been the same each year since I began weight training in 1956 at age 14: begin training with a purpose in January after putting on excess bodyfat over the Christmas holidays. It's an easy program to start with, training every other day or training after two days rest. The important element of beginning a new program is regularity in your training. By following *Diaries* day by day you will get the program and structure of the beginning phases of training. This rhyme sticks in my mind, and helps me remember the first workout:

JANUARY 1

FIRST WORKOUT

Memories of workouts great
motivates me to get in shape
and grows into a sense of urgency
that results in a brief workout with a friend.
Like birds we were free and had fun
the pump was on me:
Leg extension
leg curl
leg press
and Leg Blaster squats
one set of 10 reps
then calf raises three varieties:
standing
seated
and donkeys
doing reps close to failure
getting a burn
flames we could almost see.
Now it's my turn.
After resting one minute we did upper body:
front pulldown
incline presses
low cable row
shrugs
curls
and pressdowns
Finished with 100 ab reps
and aerobics alike:
knee-up
crunch
and 20 minutes stationary bike.

REMINISCENCE MEDITATING

Woke up this morning and the unburned smell of crusty old logs in the fireplace
made me think of when I bought a Christmas gift for my father long ago at age 10.
A 59-cent hammer and other cheap tools certainly were nothing he could use.
He was an electrician and got mad at me for spending his hard earned money
so I went out and climbed my cherry tree and gazed in the sky.
Now in meditation listening to the sounds of Chopin's melodies floating by and in my
imagination attach my body's fatigue to a rainbow of sound soaring in the sky and trade
the tension stored in my thigh for peaceful oblivion. Soreness hit today. I'm not used to feeling my body this way for some time now. After meditation I did my 10 favorite stretches,
holding each one for 20 seconds without bouncing. Then ate breakfast of a tangerine,
amino acids, vitamins, minerals, enzymes, and two soft boiled eggs on a rye cracker and
a cup of decaffeinated coffee.

WORKOUT 2

Today I train with a client and must admit that even though I feel rested I'm looking forward to the good feeling after my workout more than actually doing it. With a workout partner, the routine is to alternate sets: you do 20 sets, then I do 10. This second workout is the same as the first except we add more ab work and aerobics. Concentrating, we pack more workout into less time and finish our workout at 11:59.

leg extension
10 reps
leg curl
10 reps
leg press
10 reps
Leg Blaster squats
10 reps
standing calf raises
15 reps
seated calf raises
15 reps
donkey calf raises
15 reps

UPPER BODY
front pulldown
10 reps
incline presses
10 reps
low cable row
10 reps
shrugs
10 reps
curls
10 reps
pressdowns
10 reps
dumbbell fly
10 reps

ABS
hanging knee ups
two sets of 25 reps
abdominal crunches
two sets of 25 reps
stationary bike
20 minutes

BREAKFAST

Up at the crack of dawn, I meditate for 20 minutes by visualizing a huge heart on my chest and putting the people, animals, and things I appreciate most inside it. This morning Christine and my dog Tyler make it inside before this hairy exercise machine is pawing at my study room door with leash in his mouth and we go for a 25 minute walk. An early morning breakfast was filled with fragrance of a fuchsia rosebud fused between two oranges with the scent of Kenya coffee, decaf for Christine, banana sandwiches on two slices whole grain toast apiece. Glasses of water wash down vitamins, minerals, and amino acids between bites of food. Tyler brings the newspaper to Christine who reads the news and we visualize what is going on in the world today. After breakfast, business beckons me to start my day.

W O R K O U T   3

My whole body is too much for me to confront in one workout, so I split my routine in half and train only *upper body-abs* today. Two sets of each exercise: a warm-up set and then add weight for the second set. I combine two exercises into super-sets, that is, two exercises are done one immediately after the other then rest and stretch for 15 seconds after each super-set. Slow negatives are in order: one rep every six seconds; a two-second positive and four-second negative (return to starting position). Using push/pull super-sets economizes the workout time:

{ **dumbbell front press**
{ **front pulldown**
{ **incline dumbbell press**
{ **low cable row**
{ **dumbbell fly or pec dec**
{ **parallel dips**
{ **dumbbell pullover**
{ **dumbbell rear deltoid raises**
  one-arm side cable raise
  (two nonstop sets with each arm)
{ **triceps pressdown**
{ **face down incline dumbbell curl**
{ **one-arm dumbbell triceps extension**
{ **one-arm dumbbell concentration curl**
{ **barbell reverse curl**
{ **barbell wrist curl**

   ABS
{ **hanging knee up**
{ **abdominal crunch**

LUNCH

Relaxing in traction after a stretching work out
the wild beast roaring in my stomach said "time to eat."
Six chicken breasts thawing make poultry to cook
in a saucepan with a little jalapeño
a teaspoon of olive oil and four ounces chianti vino.
Pasta in water's boiling force draining noodles al dente
mixed with tomato sauce low sodium of course
are cooked all together
we ate it with gusto
everything was so tender.

PAYING NO ATTENTION TO PAIN

Shivering inside, a cold morning militia of pain
skating by on rollerblades stabs the back of my mouth.
The throbbing molar gives me good reason not to work out.
Three hours at two dentists helped ease my pain
but by the time I got home it was back again.
So I did a light/sound program riding the stationary bike
pulses of 30 hertz up to 40 then down for 20 minutes and pain's gone again.
Light sound entrainment enveloped my attention
hurts became hertz.
We are our attention, we become what we think.
What is my mind? It's what's on my mind.
Where is my mind? It's stored all through my body by chance
and in the hurt of my tooth as light/sound entrainment trick my body
into trance and I forget what now seems like a painful illusion.

WORKOUT 4

My leg workout begins with an early morning mile walk on the treadmill followed by a set of 12 reps then 10 reps of the following exercises:

leg extension
  12 reps then 10
leg curl
  12 reps then 10
leg press
  12 reps then 10 each
Leg Blaster squats
  12 reps then 10 each

  CALVES (do reps by holding at the top of the
  movement for a count of five)
standing calf raise
seated calf raise
donkeys

  ABS
ab crunches
hanging knee ups
  both two sets of 25 reps
seated twist
  100 reps

I finish before 8:00 A.M., followed by a breakfast of oatmeal, coffee, and two poached eggs.

SHOPPING FOR IDENTITY

Went shopping today and realized we live through what we purchase.
I identify or say "I" to whatever I buy.
I am that and then some
anything I want I buy I become.
Went to bed around midnight woke at 5:30 and practiced
a conscious six to seven A.M. reverie enveloped in a magical body of light.
Listening to my internal muse sing me sex to heaven harmony
humming octave of middle C in delight.
Swirling pink noise ideas are perhaps nature's bribe
to lure me away from what's missing in my being.
Shadow archetype left over evolutionary beast
living in my gut also abides in the creative crystal ball of light
crack between worlds of quartz red-orange glowing lava sun
pulsating a million hertz and then some.

W O R K O U T   5

Remembering how important it is to stretch after every exercise and that stretching is a great workout in itself, today I start using the three-way split paradigm where Day One is *back-biceps-forearms*. Together these pulling muscles work just fine. Day Two is legs: calves and thighs, and Day Three for the pushing muscles I design a session about chest shoulders and triceps with a little ab work and aerobics at the end of every workout.

Today's workout is day one:

BACK
two-arm lat stretch
15 seconds (holding steady without bounce)
front pulldown
two sets of 10 reps with slow negatives
low cable row
two sets of 10 reps with slow negatives
dumbbell shrug
two sets of 10 reps with slow negatives
one-arm dumbbell row
two sets of 10 reps with slow negatives
one-arm lat stretch
two sets of 10 reps with slow negatives

BICEPS
concentration dumbbell curl
two sets of 10 reps with slow negatives
cable curl on the preacher bench
two sets of 10 reps with slow negatives
incline dumbbells curled face down
two sets of 10 reps with slow negatives

FOREARMS
barbell
two sets with 80 pounds for 10 reps with slow negatives
reverse curl
two sets of 10 reps with slow negatives
wrist curl
two sets of 10 reps with slow negatives
grippers

the same ab work as last time

rowing machine
500 meters

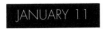

DAY OF PAIN

Returned to the dentist who said it was OK to wear my Mind/Muscle™ machine
while he drilled and x-rayed. With several Novocain injections
my mouth was numb as could be.
The sight and sound of nine to 13 hertz frequencies
made this otherwise aversive session into pain wave entrainment
the entire two hours. It was more like entertainment.
But when I got home the throbbing began
so I did more entrainment with even higher frequencies again.
Subsiding, the pain lay waiting to gain my attention with any physical exertion,
so I watch a little TV and then before bed take three milligrams of melatonin,
fall asleep easily and experience resplendent dreams...
later awake and feel better again.
Keeping busy with work all day made me realize
the experience of pain depends upon my attention to it.
It was best to pay attention to something else.

EARTHQUAKE

The next day while still asleep, the earth rumbled at 3:39 A.M.
to the Richter scale tune of 5.5 in what seemed like a night of terror.
But I fell asleep again dreaming golden white light images with
crimson tinges
engulfing my whole being. Perhaps the quake was the earth's
refrain—
an omen of the last of my pain.
Cautious, I make a decision not to train today,
and read most of the day instead.
Went out for an early dinner with Christine at 3 P.M. and
had a tossed salad, baked potato, steamed broccoli,
and a 12-ounce sirloin steak medium rare.

W O R K O U T   6

Feeling an impulse to do a one-hour *leg* workout, I'm in the gym by 3 P.M. ready to start. Today I use the Leg Blaster, my own invention, to make squats and calf raises easier.

leg curl
  two sets of 10 reps
leg extension
  two sets of 10 reps
Leg Blaster squats
  12 reps with 100 then 120 pounds
calf raises with Leg Blaster
  two sets of 20 reps with 130 pounds holding each rep
  for five seconds at the top

treadmill
  10 minutes
stationary bike
  10 minutes

  ABS
hanging knee up
crunch

seated twist
  more reps than before

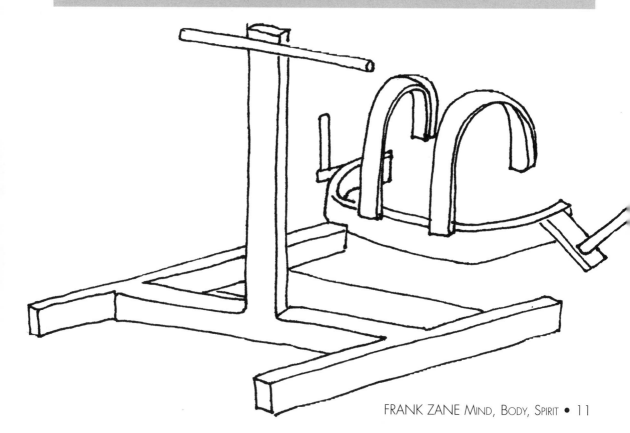

OPALS IN AUSTRALIA

Mr. Olympia Contest in Sydney, 1980
opals bought in Australia
what haunts me is the memory of fear
beginning the end of my competitive bodybuilding career.
Arnold training advice
taught me competition's strategy not friendship
healing old wounds became a 1981 contest sacrifice
came back 200 pounds strong and massive
bigger than ever in 1982
with 19-inch arms impressive
that bench pressed over
300 pounds with a 10 second negative.
Pressing 10 reps with 90-pound dumbbells
on the 70-degree incline was commonplace
but all this was only good enough for second place
London Mr. Olympia
what a disgrace.
Drew lucky number seven in 1983
and placed only fourth in Munich, Germany
as defined as could be,
the best I could do weighing 183.
Later ate sausage drank Octoberfest beer
then went to Italy
and changed 600 dollars into one million lire.
We couldn't spend it all in the streets of Florence.
Millionaires buying memories then
dashed hope washed away
in the wine of bodybuilding oblivion amen.
Woke up nine years later at age 50
got into best shape since competition
proving myself by dropping to 170.
Wrote Fabulously Fit Forever.
Expanded bodybuilding as developmental psychology.
Now four years older with lower back pain
I overcome inertia and
start training hard again.

WORKOUT 7

"**N**o I won't; yes I will" rage the voices of my mind. Call them subpersonalities, still they're nothing more than different aspects of me, until an itching in my chest symbolizes my real desire to train harder. Today's workout is *chest-shoulders-triceps*. I waited an hour after breakfast then started:

dumbbell front press
  two sets of 10 reps
pec deck
  two sets of 10 reps
30-degree incline dumbbell press
  two sets of 10 reps
dumbbell pullover
  two sets of 10 reps
parallel dips
  two sets of 12 reps
rear deltoid raises
  two sets of 12 reps with 20-pound dumbbells
dumbbell extension
  two sets of 10 reps with 30 pounds
side cable raises
  two sets of 10 reps with 30 pounds
pressdown
  two sets of 10 reps with 65 pounds
pronated dumbbell raises to the side
  two sets of 10 reps with 15 pounds

Finally, I do the usual abs and aerobics.

MY CHURCH

After meditating my eyes open to a warm morning
of glowing golden brown mountains with patches of dark
evergreen that contrast the glow of an amber porch light left on all night.
Balmy zephyr winds sing a hymn through the open window
in the church behind my gym filled with precious memories:
four bows for archery that shot aluminum arrows with wings
Casio keyboard resting on a wooden bench dearly carved by Dave Draper,
it sings, this wood from the old Santa Monica Pier.
Twin mahogany tables hold a warm lamp glowing bold
bought at Angel View Thrift mart a real bargain, late at night
it really looks smart and lights Christine's magnificent photos
in the San Bernardino national forest. Sri Chinmoy's champion tribute supreme
lifts up the world with oneness heart chorus. Wall hanging tanka bought in Belgium
for 35,000 francs in 1979 after winning Mr. Olympia the third and final time
when we walked the streets of Brugge feeling free buying real Tibetan art.
In a shop called De jonk a ree I offered an old fart $110 for a reclining deity
this price was his best, but Christine returned later and gave him American Express.
Now this Buddha watches me as we watch TV.

W O R K O U T   8

With body still in resonation with after images from 50 minutes of light sound meditation, the desire to work out bloomed into a workout plan after my Chocolate whey protein breakfast with strawberries and a teaspoon of smart powder or psyllium and one gram of the amino acid L-Glutamine. The meal fills my stomach and becomes training energy with ease. I write for two hours then hit the gym for a *back-bicep-forearms-abs* workout. The thought crossed my mind that bodybuilding changed ideas after 1979 when the monster trend came back again.

dumbbell front press
  two sets of 10 reps
pec deck
  two sets of 10 reps
30-degree incline dumbbell press
  two sets of 10 reps
dumbbell pullover
  two sets of 10 reps
dip machine
  two sets of 10 reps with 150 pounds
rear deltoid raises
  two sets of 10 reps with 20 pounds

one-arm dumbbell extension
  two sets of 10 reps with 30 pounds
one-arm side cable raises
  two sets of 10 reps with 300 pounds
{ **pressdown**
  two sets of 10 supersetted with
pronated dumbbell raises to the side

  ABS AEROBICS EXERCISES
leg raise,
  two sets of 25 reps

SANDWICH

In the waning moonlit night Castor and Pollux point to the tram light above Palm Springs shining brightly in the middle of the Western sky. Banana walnut sandwich is our breakfast vegetarian treat with whole grain sunflower seed bread from a new bakery in town. After breakfast I spend a half hour in meditation in a mental exercise I call contemplating noticeable sameness. During this time new ideas abound so I write it all down. Who really knows if this stuff is poetry or prose? Manifestation creation relaxation resonation elation splendor glowing I feel a wonderful sensation as the words keep flowing and I feel my muscles growing.

W O R K O U T   9

An hour past breakfast I know it's time to begin today's *leg* workout with sore-ness subsiding feeling a little chill that went away with a five-minute warm-up walk on the treadmill.

leg extension
leg curl
  both three sets for 10 reps (a one leg back and one leg up stretch between sets increases flexibility)
leg press
  12 reps then 10 reps with 20 pounds added
Leg Blaster squats
  12 reps with 125 pounds and 10 reps with 145 pounds
hip machine
  two sets of 12 reps

  CALVES (holding each rep five seconds at the top)
leg press calf raises
  15 reps
seated calf raise
  15 reps
donkeys
  15 reps
calf stretch

  ABS
hanging knee up
crunches
  both four sets of 25 reps
one-arm cable crunch
  both arms 50 reps
seated twist
  50 reps
stationary bike
  20 minutes

DREAMS

Dark frosty morning am I dreaming or not?
Reminds me of dark bleak frostier mornings in Pennsylvania
where tire tracks in the snow trace a cold winter mountain road
I know what three feet of deep, deep snow is like
as the night's winds blow into the valley's sleeping absolution.
I awake to this dream fragment that seems like
an unfinished solution to unresolved incidents past
that demand closure and completion.
I'm beginning to develop dream lucidity
by waking up in my dream while still asleep
and taking control of my dreams.
But this ability was short lived
and the harder I tried to wake up while still asleep
all I got was deeper sleep and my lower back hurt.
So after five hours in bed I began arising early to meditate instead.
Now instead of dreaming out of control, meditation comes easily
with mind awake and body asleep I tap into creativity.

WORKOUT 10

After a day of rest, I shift to a *chest-shoulder-tricep* workout remembering to focus on getting the best possible pump. Just in time for my workout the mail arrived with a device called "shoulder horn" to strengthen my rotator cuff. It will allow me to do external rotation with 15-pound dumbbells isolating the teres minor and infraspinatus muscles.

doorway stretch
15 seconds

dumbbell front press
really slow—as long as 10 seconds—negatives

incline dumbbell press
12 reps then increase the weight a little and do 10 reps

pec deck
12 reps then increase the weight a little and do 10 reps

dips
12 reps then increase the weight a little and do 10 reps

pullovers
12 reps then increase the weight a little and do 10 reps

rear delt machine
12 reps then 10, increasing the weight 10 pounds on the second set

triceps pressdown
12 reps then 10, increasing the weight 10 pounds on the second set

one-arm dumbbell tricep extension
12 then 10 reps

one-arm dumbbell side raises
12 then 10 reps

For abdominal variety, I do 20 minutes of ab-aerobics by combining treadmill, hanging knee-ups, bike, crunches, rowing, and seated twist.

WORKOUT 11

Feeling sore all over, I trained *abs and aerobics:*

hanging knee-ups
abdominal crunches
  both three sets of 30 to 40 reps
one-arm cable crunches
  three sets of 25

After 10 minutes on the treadmill (walking at 3.3 miles per hour), I watched a kaleidoscopic light show through closed eyelids wearing my Mind/Muscle™ machine while riding the recumbent stationary bike at a cadence of 90 for 20 minutes.

DEATH OF WINTER

It was a very cold day when my brother called to tell me
my Mother passed away. With remorse
I made reservations for the funeral in Edwardsville, Pa.
This sunless overcast morning I worked hard the entire day
mourning to catch a plane to New York, a bus to Pennsylvania
and bury my Mother. That evening's six P.M. dusk in Palm Springs
revealed cloud forms in the shape of a luminous silver blue whale
with an eye of Venus and a crescent moon's smile swimming
my mom over Mount San Jacinto with wings
where the tramlight at the top said go
straight to the Pure Western Paradise, glad
joining her was a school of whales
waiting at the peak taught by my Dad gone 26 years.
My parents united at last this way
with the moon setting behind the snowy white spires.
Mom lived two weeks past her 81st birthday
one year more than the Buddha
compassion lives forever and I pray to God, Amen.

PLANE, BUS, FUNERAL

Tuesday traveled all day:
Palm Springs to Dallas to New York to PA
On the way from LaGuardia Airport cried
feeling very sad at times thinking of how my Mother died
crying absolved a little grief.
Wednesday, at 8:30 sharp, my brother picked me up at my hotel
to go to the funeral of my Mother. She hadn't felt well
falling, breaking her hip once, then another
time in pain bed-ridden, her life a living hell
it took six feet of snow melting fast
from 60-degree temperatures and rain, the Susquehanna River swelled
fearing a flood, Mom was evacuated to higher ground
while the river crested one foot below the top of the dike
100,000 people returned home, Wilkes-Barre saved, water retired
and my Mom returned to her bed at Dorrance Manor
and at 2:30 A.M., expired.
Now gazing at her in a coffin of radiant golden splendor
place my copper hematite ring on her right forefinger
and a Lapis bracelet on her wrist
black diamond hematite alive sparkles bright
alive she helped me pump iron right
Sutras say the ground in the Pure Land's made of Lapis Lazulli
Hematite black like Pennsylvania's coal of anthracite
deep blue Lapis Pure Earth, Heavenly
Rain driving to the cemetery
carrying Mom's casket crying
oceans of tears flooding into her grave
we gave, my brother and me, each a flower
atop her golden earth capsule
raining still, the Reverend willed final words of power
over death, my Mother laid to rest
her soul free eternally.
Now looking out my window at a winter landscape bleak
black barren trees among white snowy patches
reflecting sorrow my earth feels weak
limited toward her end but blessed
My Mother is now limitless.

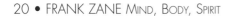

APPLE TREE OF LIFE

Last night I lay thinking
of my home in Palm Springs
where huge tamarisk branches grow
like a pine weed of the desert
that never sleeps and grows forever.
Cut, this tree always comes back
long straight branches lying on the sod
elegant trim spears
thrown and stuck in the mud.
Buried garden center
our departed dog Apple
long tall beautiful white
Royal Standard Poodle
has grown into a tree
high in the sand
her slender trunk stands
not a bend and
long tall leafy branches send
Apple loving essence
to fertile soil of heaven's
angelic pure land.
Then dusk's reddish amber crack
attracts my sight
between blue azure mountains
and grey layered clouds at twilight
diffuse headlights glowing north
on Pennsylvania route 315
perhaps the most magnificent sunset
I've ever seen
as arctic cold blows open my door
can't ignore the white column banks
oozing from cliffs they form white stalactites
below dark bare winter tree shanks.
Life's about the living
like the weather it will change
tomorrow everything will be different, again.

W O R K O U T   1 2

Struggling with sadness, I hum a hymn and force myself to train at a local gym determined this **back-bicep-forearms** workout won't be in vain. And so it began:

front pulldown
12 reps with 150 pounds then 10 with 160
cable crossover behind neck
40 pounds for 20 reps then 50 pounds for 15 reps
interjecting two-arm lat stretch between sets

after a quick drink of water:

low cable row
140 pounds then 150 for 10 reps

After lat stretching, I cut my workout short.

W O R K O U T   1 2   1 / 2

Half a workout is better than none in order to finish what I started yesterday:

rowing
500 meters in three minutes
close grip pulldown
140 pounds then 150 for 10 reps
dumbbell shrugs
65 pounds for 20 reps
one-arm lat stretch
with each arm, 15 seconds

BICEPS AND FOREARMS
face down incline dumbbell curls
27.5 pounds for 10 reps
preacher cable curl
80 pounds for 10 reps
wrist curl
60-pound barbell for 15 reps
repeat this same tri-set again with five pounds more
on each exercise

I rested between sets for a minute, then did ab work same as before.

LEAVING PENNSYLVANIA

Light blue pink strata squeeze dark mountains between headlights
streaking through a frigid morning of 11 degrees
leaving Wilkes Barre at 7:30 A.M. on a Martz Trailways bus trip.
In the back of the bus I sit watching snow speckled slag heaps of coal
embedded white birch trees amidst black arbor thin shadows
and evergreen trees conical symmetry of late January in the Poconos.
Arrive in New York City in a few hours been here often, who knows
how many times, a pity it's so freakin' cold, the wind blows
shivering from a wind chill of minus 10 degrees
walking city streets below freezing, I sneeze
looking for a music store to buy a harmonica I'm sad and still sore
that last workout feels like the 1970s in Santa Monica.
playing sad songs to myself and more
finding two in keys of C and G, can't wait to explore
Bach's Brandenburg Concertos.
Hiking to Wolfe's Restaurant on 57th Street
order a roast beef sandwich and eat, sustaining myself
stomach full, complete for the cab ride to LaGuardia
catching the 2:45 P.M. flight to Palm Springs, California.
Now five days past Mother's funeral, still can't forget it
watching myself feeling hopeless and pathetic
remorse and sadness will pass
if I let it go its own way and find others to prey on
hope someday I'll die in a noble way.
Is death all I have to look forward to? Can't say.
There must be more, praying, fall asleep on the plane, snore
awake in Palms Springs warm, stretch, shake
realize it won't take an earthquake
to make sure of the future.
I resolve to have faith.

BACK HOME

Waking up the next day
wondering will jet lag prevent me from
   training today?
Better to err on the conservative side — I'd
   force myself to train

but here my heart won't abide with this
   idea.
Ambivalently planning tomorrow I'll train.
If I had two or three grams of L-tryptophane
I'd sleep and ease my pain.

W O R K O U T   1 3

Feeling stronger after a day's rest, I know it's best to work *thighs* and *calves* today.

leg extension
   140 pounds for 12 reps
leg curl
   80 pounds for 12 reps, followed by leg back and leg
   up stretch
leg extension
   150 pounds for 10 reps
leg curl
   90 pounds for 10 reps and stretch again
leg press
   200 pounds for 12 reps and 220 pounds for 10 reps
Leg Blaster squats
   140 pounds for 12 reps and 150 for 10
hamstring stretching
hip machine
   12 reps with 90 pounds
one leg standing leg curl
   12 reps with 40 pounds
hip machine
   10 reps with 100 pounds
one leg standing leg curl
   10 reps with 60 pounds
standing calf raise
   two sets of 15 reps with 150 pounds, holding each
   rep five seconds at the top
donkeys
   15 reps
seated calf raises
   15 reps

   ABS
knee ups
   two sets of 30 reps
crunches
   two sets of 30 reps
one-arm cable crunch
   two sets of 30 reps

Ten minutes later I had amino acids and a peach.

THE PAIN OF TRAINING

My neck hurts
suddenly I'm feeling quite well
my knee creaks
can't figure why I'm still feeling swell
my groin groans
but am I happier than hell?
My lower back's impaired
here optimism dwelled,
my shoulders suffer, diffused by the knell
of the local church bell,
my elbow's injured
but not enough to make me yell,
my tricep's been tricked
by close grip bench press with a heavy barbell,
my trapezius is taut
but must pump up to excel,
my tooth throbs
won't ease the pain with Zinfandel,
my forearm's harm'd
while blood rushes to every muscle cell,
my knuckle's constrained
so copper rings I wear,
my head quakes
and casts a magic spell,
my ankle aches
but excuses won't sell,
my wrist is wrenched
instead I'll use a dumbbell,
my hamstring's pulled
so I squat only to parallel,
my butt moans
at least it doesn't smell,
my back complains
my wife says "do tell,"
my neck's still stiff
stressed at work from personnel,
but despite the pain I still train
inside you probably can't tell
pain once identified
wanes farewell.

WORKOUT 14

As the violet pink dawn settled into a grey morning, I was anxious to get to my workout. But first I sit for 20 minutes and have some peppermint tea, amino acids, and a whole grain muffin. And after a 25-minute meditation, I begin the *chest-shoulders-triceps-abs* workout with

doorway stretch
30-degree incline barbell presses
  100 pounds for 12 reps, 120 for 10 with two-second
  positive and four-second negative
70-degree incline dumbbell press
  45 pounds and 50 pounds for two sets of 10 reps
doorway stretch
  15 seconds
pec deck
  10 reps with 115 and 130 pounds
dip machine
  10 reps with 150 and 160 pounds
pullover machine
  140 and 150 pounds for 12 reps then 10
rear delt machine
  10 reps with 100 pounds, 10 with 110

  TRICEPS AND DELTS
one-arm dumbbell extension
  two sets of 10 reps with 30 pounds
one-arm dumbbell side raise
  two sets of 10 reps with 20 pounds

Finally, 15 minutes more ab work as in the previous workout.

MY DOG TYLER

Dusk's full moon
peeping through olive trees ripe
Tyler poolside at twilight
hot soup as dark approaches
wonder if he might
grow even more
a great dog, friendly and bright
full of unconditional positive regard
for me, he doesn't bite
barks at voices in the night
causing a fright, I'm sure
and brings Christine
the newspaper in bed at daylight.
Chasing five feline brothers

he breaks up a cat fight.
I'm off to L.A. this morning
he waits at the gate light
my Forrest Gump of a dog
there he is in my headlights.
At the end of the day
boomerangs I swear
he loves to play
catching them in mid-air
Tyler's really into being a dog
following me everywhere
I'm sure glad
this caramel lab-chow-rotweiler-doberman
calls me his dad.

THE DOUBLE

All beings have a double
but a warrior learns to be aware of this dual existence.
One aspect is our visible appearance, the ego we know.
The other invisible image lives in a world of dreams,
a witness of brighter rendition doubling the visible ego
this genius who watches is the supreme self who waits.
About this double the ancient Upanishads say:
Like two golden birds on the selfsame tree
Intimate friends the ego and the self,
comrades inseparable dwell in the same body.
The ego eats the sweet and sour fruits of the tree of life
while the self looks on in detachment without eating,
skipping pleasure and pain is no sacrifice.
In the secret cave of the heart these two are seated by life's fountain.
Ego drinks the sweet and bitter right from the start,
liking the sweet, hating the bitter, ego's not too smart.
The supreme self drinks of the same stuff
neither liking nor disliking isn't tough
while the ego gropes in darkness
the self lives in brilliant diamond light hewn from the rough.
Lord of the chariot is the self.
The body is the chariot itself.
Discriminating intellect is charioteer with the mind as reins we hold dear
the horses are the five senses traveling down the road of selfish desires.
When the self is mistaken for the body, mind and senses,
enjoying pleasure and suffering sorrow become what life's about.
There's more to it than that say those who know.
Burning in the heart enshrined is a flame without smoke.
Ruler of past and future time right here
today and tomorrow always the same
to know the self is to go beyond fear.

WORKOUT 15

Today's *back-biceps-forearms* workout, which I completed in an hour and 20 minutes, began with two minutes of warm-up rowing and 15 seconds two-arm lat stretch holding the knob of a door.

front pulldown
10 reps with 160 pounds, then 10 reps at 170 with slow negatives throughout and at the top of the movement not locking out

low cable row
10 reps with 150 and 160 pounds

one-arm cable row
two sets of 12 reps at 90 pounds, with a one-arm lat stretch between each set

shrugs
two sets of 15 reps with 65-pound dumbbells

I take a break to eat a small tangerine

BICEPS
face down incline dumbbell curl
two sets of 10 reps with 25 pounds

preacher cable curl
two sets of 10 reps with 70 pounds

face up 45-degree curl on the incline bench
two sets of 10 reps with 22.5 pounds

FOREARMS
barbell reverse curl
two sets of 10 reps with 70 pounds

barbell wrist curl
two sets of 20 reps for 80 pounds

squeezing two grippers
two sets of 20 reps, after which I had to shake my hands out a few minutes

ABS (three tri-sets)
{
hanging knee ups
30 reps
crunches
30 reps
seated twist
30 reps
}

rowing machine
500 meters

DOCTOR DREAM

A doctor in my dream said "I would like to have more patients.
I need patients to be successful."
Awakening, realizing I need more patience too.
Its true, dreams can be fun to find out their meaning.
This dream was a play on words, or pun
the language of unconscious mind.

WORKOUT 16

A *leg* workout is on my calendar today.

leg extension
 20 reps
leg curl
 20 reps
leg press
 20 reps
Leg Blaster squats
 20 reps
hip machine
 20 reps
one-legged curl
 20 reps
treadmill
 five minutes
stationary bike
 five minutes

 CALVES (holding reps for five seconds at the top)
standing calf raises
seated calf raises
donkeys

NOCTURNAL WIND

Swift windstorm delivers a merciless 50 mile an hour massage
to the huge eucalyptus trees nearby when
suddenly the wind is replaced by a warm cool breeze
wafting through my window with ease
and it's quiet again before the 5 A.M. hour.
Out of black vastness shines the power
of the constellation Gemini in the western sky
turning on my morning lamp lines from T.S. Eliot's
Four Quartets reminds me why
simply put, to get where I'm not
to go to my goal, I must travel the way
where there is no ecstasy only ignorance on the spot,
dispossession preceedes possession
and all I know and own is not a lot.

WORKOUT 17

The four days that have past since the last upper body workout have given my shoulders a good rest. So now I'm ready to test *chest-delts-triceps*.

70-degree incline dumbbell front press
  12 reps with 45 pounds, then 10 reps with 50 pounds
  doing ultra slow 10-second negatives
30-degrees incline dumbbell press
  12 reps with 55 pounds then 10 reps with 60 pounds;
  working in doorway stretch with both of these front
  delt/upper pec movements
dumbbell fly
  two sets of 10 reps with 35 pounds
parallel dip
  two sets of 10 reps with bodyweight
dumbbell pullover
  two sets of 10 reps with 50 pounds

  DELTS AND TRICEPS
one-arm dumbbell tricep extension
  30 pounds for two sets of 10 reps
side cable raise
  30 pounds for two sets of 12 reps
pressdown
  holding a hard lockout at the end for two sets of 10 reps
pronated dumbbell side raises
  15 pounds for two sets of 12 slow reps

Finally, I do the usual ab work and 12 minutes
of treadmill.

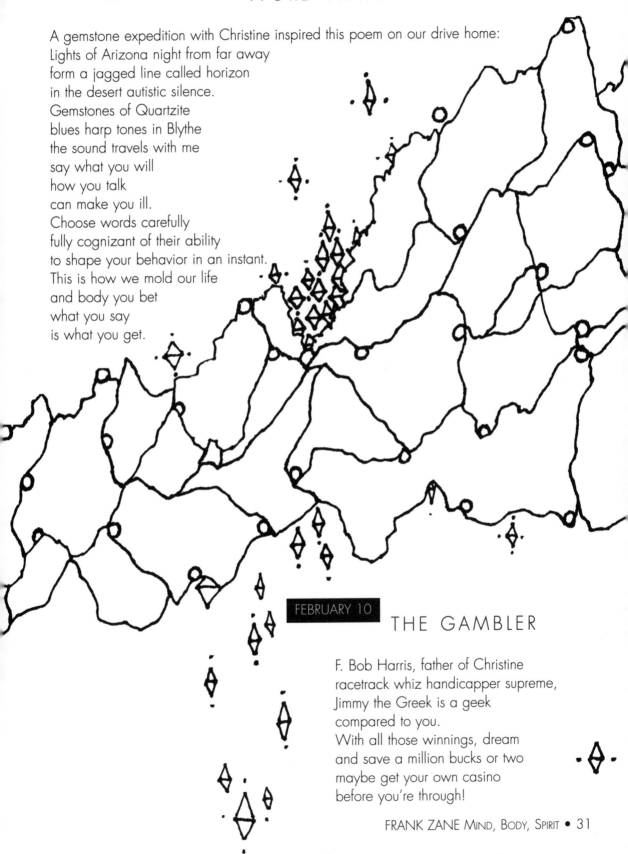

WORD TRAVEL

A gemstone expedition with Christine inspired this poem on our drive home:
Lights of Arizona night from far away
form a jagged line called horizon
in the desert autistic silence.
Gemstones of Quartzite
blues harp tones in Blythe
the sound travels with me
say what you will
how you talk
can make you ill.
Choose words carefully
fully cognizant of their ability
to shape your behavior in an instant.
This is how we mold our life
and body you bet
what you say
is what you get.

THE GAMBLER

F. Bob Harris, father of Christine
racetrack whiz handicapper supreme,
Jimmy the Greek is a geek
compared to you.
With all those winnings, dream
and save a million bucks or two
maybe get your own casino
before you're through!

W O R K O U T   1 8

Well developed latissimus dorsi will take a long time and a lot of work to build. This 1976 workout was one of my very best. But if I did it today, I'd do only *two sets of each* exercise and *use two-thirds of the weight* with *more stretching in between sets:*

barbell rowing
   eight sets, doing 10 reps beginning with 110, 130, 150, 160, 170, 180, 190, and 200 pounds
one-arm dumbbell row
   10 reps with 100, 110, and 120 pounds
behind the neck pulldown
   10 reps with 190, 200, and 210 pounds
low cable row
   10 reps with 180, 190, and 200 pounds
shrugs
   three sets of 12 reps with 100-pound dumbbells

   BICEPS
alternate dumbbell
   three sets of 10 reps with 55 pounds
curls on the preacher bench
   100-pound barbell for three sets of 10 reps
one-arm concentration curl
   three sets of 10 reps with 45-pound dumbbell, slowly let down

   FOREARMS (three supersets)
{ **barbell reverse curl**
   100 pounds for high reps
  wrist curl
   100 pounds for high reps

MY MOTHER-IN-LAW

Josephine R. Harris, Christine's mamma
inconceivably good at the drama of selling cosmetics
improving local aesthetics
and will give more than her two cents
to help clients vent the slightest odor
which becomes sweet violet.
People come from everywhere
to hear Ms. Josephine bare
her wonderful secret scent
on all who have spent
more than their rent on
Oscar de La Renta.

W O R K O U T   1 9

An hour following a breakfast of two slices whole grain toast and three soft boiled eggs, I thought about getting ready for my *leg* workout.

CALVES
leg press machine calf raise
15 reps with 200, then 220 pounds
donkeys
250 pounds for 15 reps, holding each rep five seconds at the top
seated calf raise
100 pounds for 15 reps, holding each rep five seconds at the top

THIGHS
leg curl
two sets of 10 reps with 90 pounds, which contracts calves as well as hamstrings through the entire movement
leg extension
two sets with 150 pounds for 10 reps
Leg Blaster squat
two sets with 150 pounds for 10 reps
hip machine
12 reps with 90 pounds, then 10 with 100, one-leg back stretch between sets

AB-AEROBICS (one minute on each exercise going around the following circuit twice)
leg raise
crunches
treadmill
arm cable crunch
rowing
stationary bike

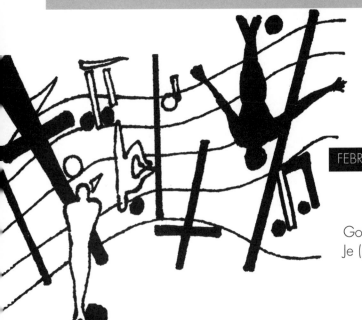

PRAYER SONG
(with musical notes)

God (c) sin (f) Christ (d) Zen (g)
Je (g) sus (f) heart (c) A (d) men (c)

W O R K O U T   2 0

Using my Mind/Muscle™ machine seems to turn me into a radio tuned to 11 hertz and "I will get the best *chest-shoulder-triceps* workout yet," I say to myself. I warm up pushing and pulling with my hands only on the Schwinn Airdyne for one minute.

UPPER PECS
five-foot Olympic barbell press on a 30-degree incline
12 reps with 110 pounds and 10 reps with 130 for each set

doorway stretch for 15 seconds
70-degree dumbbell press
45 and 50 pounds for 12 then 10 reps

pec deck
130 and 140 pounds for 12 then 10 reps followed by more doorway stretching

parallel dips
two sets of 10 reps with bodyweight

dumbbell pullover on a 5-degree decline
two sets of 10 reps with 50 pounds

one-arm shoulder stretch
one-arm dumbbell triceps extension
two sets of 12 reps with 30 pounds

one arm side cable raise
two sets of 12 reps with 30 pounds

pressdown
two sets of nine reps for 80 pounds

rear delt machine
two sets of nine reps for 110 pounds

leg raise
two sets of 30 reps

crunch
two sets of 30 reps

seated twist
100 reps nonstop

rowing
750 meters

MIND MINE

What is the mind but memories mine
the present doesn't hesitate to pass into the past.
My mind's recollection is all reflection
days gone by, bygone days.
Looking back in my mind
remember New York City skyline
from LaGuardia seen faraway
across the fuselage of an American Airlines plane
Empire State, Chrysler building
and Wall Street towers aloft gazing through the haze
before my flight takes off reflecting on happier days
when my parents were alive.
Traveling back east, always staying on California time
everything in New York was three hours late.
Living in the past, it wasn't hard work
wishing my parents lives did last
longer, their lives make me a stronger person.

THE FIVE-DAY SEQUENCE

Feeling it's about time to
get started training a little harder
have in mind somewhat random a schedule
workouts using a five-day sequence
the same three way split as before
this time training two days in a row
then resting a day
this way I know
I will get enough rest
then train the next day
and relaxing again
on the fifth final day.
Explaining this sequence
another way, I'd say
train two days on
one off, one on, one off then
start all over again.
Tomorrow I'll train this way with a friend.

W O R K O U T   2 1

W ith elbows a little sore I warm up with two sets of 25 reps barbell wrist curl pumping up my forearms first, I get more from my *back-biceps-forearms* workout.

BACK
front pulldown
150 pounds for 12 reps, 160 for 10
cable crossover behind neck
40 and 50 pounds for 20 reps
low cable row
10 reps with 150 and 160 pounds
dumbbell shrugs
two sets of 15 reps with 70 pounds
one-arm cable row
two sets of 10 reps with 90 pounds

BICEPS
one-arm dumbbell concentration curl
two sets of 10 reps with 35 pounds, slow negatives
seated one-arm dumbbell curl
10 reps with 35, then eight reps with 40 pounds
preacher cable curl
two sets of 12 reps with 80 pounds
reverse barbell wrist curl
two sets of eight reps with 60 pounds

ABS
knee ups
two sets of 30 reps
crunches
two sets of 40 reps
rowing
500 meters

WORKOUT 22

Beginning *leg* training promptly at noon:

leg curl
  12 reps with 80 and 90 pounds
leg extension
  12 reps with 140 and 150 pounds
leg pressing
  15 reps for two sets with 220 pounds
Leg Blaster squats
  two sets of 10 reps with 100 and 120 pounds, without
  locking out, kept all the tension in the thighs
hip machine
  10 reps with 90 then 100 pounds on each leg, all the
  time doing one leg back and one leg up stretching
  between sets
standing calf raises
  two sets of 15 reps, holding each rep for five seconds
  at the top
donkeys
  two sets of 15 reps, holding each rep for five seconds
  at the top
seated raises
  two sets of 15 reps, holding each rep for five seconds
  at the top

  AB-AEROBICS (one minute on each of the following exercises, then repeating the circuit again)
12-degree incline treadmill
leg raises
recumbent stationary bike
crunches
hanging knee-up
seated twist

SOUND TABLE

Installed a Somatron sound table in my gym today
connecting it to the stereo amplifier.
I was able to hook up my Mind/Muscle™ machine
and lie down on it and listen to music massage my entire body
a total audio visual experience kinesthetic
blowing fuses with a powerful amp while playing CDs
using stronger fuses with audio tapes made relaxation a breeze
tight muscles blew off tension to my body's delight
after a few minutes thought I might relax really deep
so easily I could fall asleep so saved it for tonight.

W O R K O U T   2 3

Not locking out is essential to a chest workout because it keeps continuous tension in the pecs. Not allowing pecs to return to homeostasis while doing the set always gives me a hell of a burn. Today I'm training with a client on *chest-shoulders-triceps*. First we warm up our shoulders on the Schwinn Airdyne before we start the Day 3 workout.

70-degree dumbbell front press
followed by a doorway stretch after a set of 12 reps with 45-pounders, increasing the weight to 50-pounders for 10 reps

30-degree incline dumbbell press
50 pounds for a slow 10 reps, followed by a stretch, then 55 pounds for eight reps

dumbbell fly
two sets with 35 pounds for 12 reps

parallel dip
two sets with bodyweight for 10 reps, then one-arm shoulder stretching

dumbbell pullover
55 pounds for 12 reps, then 60 for 10

one-arm dumbbell extension
12 reps with 30 pounds, then 10 with 32.5

one-arm dumbbell side raise
two sets for 10 reps with 22.5 pounds

rear delt machine
90 pounds for 12 reps, 100 for 10

triceps pressdown
65 pounds for 12 reps, 70 for 10

rowing machine
600 meters

ABS
hanging knee-ups
crunches
one-arm cable crunch with each arm
two sets of 30 reps on each exercise

SORE, IDEAS SOAR

Temor, earthquake, I'm awake.
"Did you feel it," Christine said.
I'm sore from working out, tired lying in bed
wondering is it more important instead to get up,
write down all these words and ideas flowing into my head
when my mind starts to shout "get up feel inspired
you're forgetting a lot, don't let novel cognition expire..."
I dread to miss any more so implore my tired body to arise
and catch what's left instead—it's already 6 A.M., I write
feeling weary and cold despite blurry eyes, bleary
need glasses to find my glasses to see clearly
and write what need be said in this bodybuilding winter
full of new beginnings merge to create
the progress that becomes an early spring.
People often wonder why I get so sore
without doing more than two sets of each exercise
but it's more important to realize
not why, but how to do each movement
is really what's wise to get this effect
and how much is enough to do before you're through
working calves, abs, thighs or any other bodypart.
Several years ago it was time to
depart from conventional training ideas.
Now, the most I'll ever do is three sets of each exercise
by increasing weight and lowering reps
I know you will get a great pump
before your workout is through.

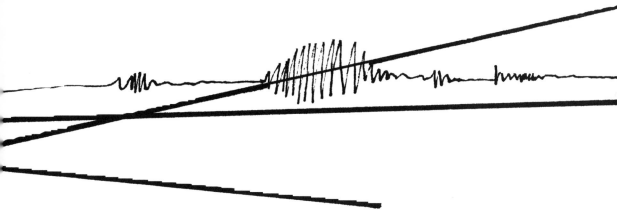

W O R K O U T   2 4

The last three good workouts under my lifting belt plus a very relaxing day of rest I am ready for an innovative *back-biceps-forearms* workout.

BACK

front pulldown
12 reps with 150 pounds, 10 for 160, eight for 170, without fully extending my arms at the top of each rep keeps all the tension in my lats, not delts; two-arm lat stretch between sets

low cable row
(with pulley three feet above the floor)
10 reps with 140 and 150 pounds as I kept doing lat stretch, adding one-arm shoulder stretch

one-arm dumbbell row
two sets of 10 reps lowering a 70-pound dumbbell all the way down interspersed with one-arm lat stretch with each arm

close grip pulldown
10 reps with 140 pounds, then 10 with 150

dumbbell shrug
two sets of 20 reps with 65 pounds

BICEPS

one-arm dumbbell concentration curl
two sets of 10 reps with 35 pounds

seated one-arm dumbbell curl
two sets of eight reps with 40 pounds

preacher cable curl
two sets of 10 reps using 80 pounds

incline dumbbell curl face down
two sets of 12 reps using 25 pounds

FOREARMS

reverse wrist curl
two sets of 10 reps with 50 pounds

barbell wrist curl
two sets of 10 reps with 70 pounds

rowed
750 meters

ABS

knee ups
crunches
both exercises for four sets of 25 reps

QUICK MEAL

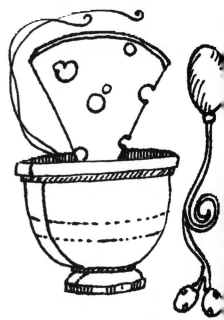

Lunch today took five minutes to prepare:
A can of fat-free vegetable soup
a can of white albacore tuna
mixed together in a bowl with jalapeño sauce
cooked in microwave for three minutes
two slices of low fat swiss cheese laid on top
gave me about 60 grams of protein
30 grams of carbohydrate and very little fat.
Quite tasty at that for a lean meal.

VARIABLE REINFORCEMENT

Woke up this morning feeling more tired than usual
so I decided to work legs tomorrow, I'm told
from learning theory and training 40 years
my conclusion is two fold:
the body thrives on routine it is clear,
appears to get used to the same thing quickly, gets old
and then stops responding, a sticking point everyone fears.
Psychological learning theory taught me
a training technique that saves me tears,
called variable schedules of reinforcement
simply stated says train an animal with rewards, where's
they're given the same amount, always the same time in between...
stop giving the rewards and the desired behavior disappears.
Now the body is like an animal in this respect
doing the same routine always the same way, it is
good at first but your body, just like the animal knows
when the reward comes, stop the reward
and the behavior won't persevere.
But reinforce the animal in variable times and amounts
and it won't figure out when the payoff is in arrears
and keeps responding, expecting the reward to appear.
It's the same with all animals, your body included
it works with workouts, food supplements
and drugs, don't be deluded, just look in the mirror
reinforce on a variable schedule, you'll keep enjoying
and you won't be excluded from the progress you're after.
You will improve even faster!

W O R K O U T   2 5

In order to catch an 11:30 A.M. plane for the Arnold Classic, I was in the gym by 8 o'clock for a giant set (more than three exercises done without stopping) for legs.

leg extension
  12 reps with 150 pounds
leg curl
  12 reps with 90 pounds
leg press
  10 reps with 220 pounds
Leg Blaster squat
  10 reps with 100 pounds
standing calf raise
  15 reps with 100 pounds
leg press calf raise
  15 reps with 220 pounds
donkeys
  15 reps with 200 pounds
seated calf raise
  15 reps with 100 pounds
knee ups
  50 reps
crunches
  50 reps

HELLO COLUMBUS

Arrived last night in Columbus, Ohio
set up my Leg Blaster booth next morning
at the Arnold Fitness Expo all day felt really excited,
wired, then crashed at my hotel, extremely tired.
Now meeting people all day long, signing autographs
and doing 50 sets of one rep on Leg Blaster squats
see old friends, reminisce, laugh
by the end of the day exhaustion sets in.
Tomorrow morning plan
to work chest shoulders triceps
on my favorite machines in Expo auditorium.

W O R K O U T 2 6

At 7:30 A.M. I start my workout with a friend in the vast expo auditorium. First, we find an upper body bike and warm up shoulders before we hike over to another booth.

30-degree incline press on the Smith machine
  12 reps with 100 pounds, 10 reps with 115
pec deck
  10 reps with 115 pounds, eight with 130
parallel dip machine
  12 reps at 150 pounds, 10 with 160
pullover machine
  10 reps with 140 pounds, 10 with 150
pressdown on lat machine
  two sets of 10 reps with 75 pounds
one-arm dumbbell triceps extension
  two sets of 10 reps with 30 pounds
one-arm dumbbell side raise
  two sets of 10 reps with 20 pounds
rear delt machine
  two sets of 12 with 90 pounds
hanging knee ups
  three sets of 30 reps

W O R K O U T 2 7

Waking up around 8 A.M., I started my Mind/Muscle™ machine meditation. After coffee, a pack of chocolate whey protein, and a banana, I gradually swallowed three liver extract, two lecithin, two biovital, and two pancreatic enzyme tablets with a diet soda throughout the meal. I was now ready for the fitness expo again with much more stamina. Arriving early at the expo, I did two supersets of leg curl and extension.

Then at my booth, I loaded up the Leg Blaster and did many sets of the erect squat and calf raises illustrating to the people coming by why it's much better to squat with upper body erect, not bending forward. This develops the thighs more and helps to avoid lower back and knee injury.

COLUMBUS — PALM SPRINGS

Left Columbus this morning on United Airlines
arriving in Chicago, catching a flight
to Palm Springs and got here three hours later, fine
it was good to be home all right
hugging Christine, dogs, petting my cats
we dined, relaxing into the night
reading, watching TV in my favorite chair, sat
thinking about whether I should train right
away tomorrow or wait at least a day at that
decided to see how I would feel waking up bright
and early the following day, not worried about getting fat
from not training, the stress of travel more than a slight
aerobic workout, forgetting about it....I took a bath
and went to bed instead.

BEAT DAY

Woke up wondering "Am I dead or alive?"
No way will I work out today.
Got the thought of training out of my head
right away and spent the day writing and reading instead.
Rilke poetry and "Desolation Angels" of Kerouac,
inspired by the great physiques
seen at the Arnold Classic.
Reading up to page 89 of "Big Sky Mind" helped me unwind
and felt just fine listening to Mozart's piano concerto nineteen
with my Mind/Muscle machine
on my Somatron sound table, lying down
conserving energy, relaxing
just enjoying the ease of things.

ABDOMINAL TRANSCENDENCE

Learned a long time ago when in doubt, don't work out,
but feeling the need to train I'm in the gym again
and decide to transcend my best recent abdominal efforts.
Had enough rest to do my best, I contend
and remember Sri Chinmoy who every day does more
in his running, one-arm lifting, bodybuilding
and now specializing like never before on abdominal training.
Everyday in his ashram gym or at the Central Queens YMCA
hundreds of situps day after day Guru's way to say
abdominals obey, fat go away obliques, intercostals,
rectus ab definition you may stay and behold
this waistline shrink to prime condition
let it be told his supreme attitude transcendental
inspires me to work harder two fold:
hanging knee up
and crunch,
abdominal training three sets of 30 each without rest
in between, always the best possible maximum burn.
Fat worn away next by one-arm cable crunches
and leg raise three supersets of 30 each in turn
breathless, no rest, sample a drink of water,
praise this Holy Example, and think of ways to finish up,
decide to include treadmill in the aerobic plan
after 30 minutes on it, can hardly stand
up lifted oneness heart prays.

W O R K O U T   2 8

My lower back and abs are sore in the morning. So I fasten body magnets in place with a velcro belt around my waist, and the pain abates during a breakfast of whey protein and fruit. I relax an hour, then warm up my lower back with

one leg up stretch
30 seconds on each leg
rowing machine
500 meters in three minutes
two-arm lat stretch
15 seconds
front pulldown using parallel grip bar
10 reps with 150, 165, then 180 pounds followed by more stretching
low cable row
10 reps with 150 and 160 pounds
shrugs
two sets of 20 reps with 65-pound dumbbells and soreness in my back disappears
one-arm rowing machine
three sets of 10 reps with 90 pounds to finish my back workout

BICEPS
seated one-arm dumbbell curl
10 reps with 30, then 35 pounds with each arm
preacher cable curl
10 reps with 80 and 90 pounds
one-arm dumbbell concentration curl
10 reps with 30 and 35 pounds on each arm

FOREARMS
reverse wrist curl with barbell
two sets of 10 reps with 60 pounds
barbell wrist curl
two sets of 15 reps with 80 pounds
grippers
20 reps squeezing out

ABS
crunches
leg raise
both two sets of 40 reps

WORKOUT 29

Today's leg workout, with 12 reps on the first sets then 10 on the second

leg curl
  80 pounds for 12 reps, then 80 for 10
leg extension
  140 pounds for 12 reps, then 150 for 10
leg press
  200 pounds for 12 reps, then 220 for 10
Leg Blaster squats
  120 pounds for 12 reps, then 140 for 10
hip machine
  90 pounds for 12 reps, then 100 for 10

  CALVES
standing calf raise
  15 reps holding five seconds at the top of each rep
leg press
  15 reps holding five seconds at the top of each rep
donkeys
  15 reps holding five seconds at the top of each rep
seated calf raise
  15 reps holding five seconds at the top of each rep

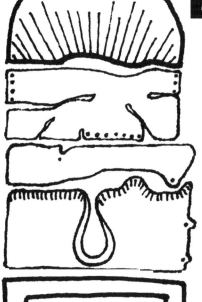

MARCH 7

NIRVANA DON'T WANNA

Mind/Muscle is not hustle but a hook to look at what is
we can't conceive or believe. We invent our perception
all the time so sit down please, meditate, contemplating
emptiness without form, sound unborn beyond conception
not realizing or knowing or wanting to know
that all that is and ever will be
is what right now is happening to me
making it all up
go on thinking there's more
but what really is
is there's nothing more
nothing beyond the door of the five senses, I find
mind making the world
world making the mind.
Is this dream stuff body an intermediate step
prerequisite before leaping into a wilderness of emptiness
quantum physics, ultimate Nirvana?
Can't say or conceive it yet, anyway.

FRANK ZANE MIND, BODY, SPIRIT • 47

W O R K O U T   3 0

With the warming weather and spring fast approaching, I feel like working out at 5 P.M. with Christine who does a half-hour on the treadmill and 15 minutes on weights. Today I will work ***chest-shoulders-triceps***.

FRONT DELTS/UPPER PECS
70-degree dumbbell front press
 two sets of 10 reps with 45 pounds
dumbbell flys
 two sets of 10 reps with 35 pounds
30-degree incline dumbbell press
 two sets of 10 reps each with 50 pounds
dumbbell pullover
 two sets of 10 reps each with 55 pounds
dips
 two sets of 12 reps then 10 reps with bodyweight
dumbbell rear deltoid raises
 two sets of 12 reps then 10 reps with 20 pounds
one-arm dumbbell tricep extension
 two sets of 10 reps with 25 pounds
side cable raise
 two sets of 10 reps with 20 pounds
rowed
 750 meters

knee ups
crunches
seated twist
 three sets of 30 reps each
treadmill
fast walking for 20 minutes

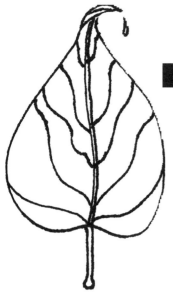

B O D H I B U I L D I N G

A friend Ken O'Neill told me the name
"Bodhibuilding," the sound of which I liked.
Bodhi is the tree the Buddha sat under to gain enlightenment.
Building is the process of creating by turning energy into matter.
Bodhi is a tree, a structure, like a building
that grows upward into the sky.
Why bodhibuilding could be called the framework I
use to turn dream stuff into a towering body,
exemplifying an enlightened self.

SPRING BREEZE

Tamarisk trees like immense desert weeds
get too close will make you wheeze
voice in the breeze says please trim these before spring.

MARCH 11

W O R K O U T   3 1

Resting two days between upper body workouts is sometimes necessary when shoulders are vigorously trained. Today my plan is to train *back-biceps-fore-arms*.

rowing
  500 meters for a warm up
front pulldown
  12, 10, and eight reps with 155, 170, and 185 pounds
low cable row
  10 reps with 155, then 165 pounds
dumbbell shrugging
  75 pounds for 10 reps, then eight reps with a five-second pause at the top of each rep
one-arm cable rowing
  two sets of 12 reps each arm with 100 pounds
facedown dumbbell incline curl
  25 pounds for 12 reps, then 30 pounds for 10 reps with each arm
one-arm dumbbell concentration curl
  two sets of 10 reps with 35 pounds

  FOREARMS
barbell reverse curl
  two sets of 20 reps with 90 pounds
barbell wrist curl
  two sets of 20 reps with 90 pounds
grippers
  25 reps, then rest

  ABS
hanging knee up
crunches
  three sets of 30 reps each
leg raise
one-arm cable crunches
  two sets of 30 reps each
stationary bicycling
  15 minutes

Christine, Christine
my wife
married me at 19
without a doubt
most significant other
in my life
lover, friend
money spender, pain mender
silver gem splendor
wonderful mother
two dogs five cats
being with her
that's enjoyment no end
arguments? quickly mend
she will freely bend
backward showing
intuition knowing
what's going
on way before me.

MARCH 13

W O R K O U T   3 2

Today I'll concentrate on *thighs*.

leg extension
  10 reps at 150 and 160 pounds
leg curl
  10 reps at 80 and 90 pounds; breathless, I rest five
  minutes
Leg Blaster squats
  20 reps with 100 pounds, then 20 with 120; after five
  minutes rest, I do 20 reps with 140 pounds

As I'm lying on the floor thinking that wasn't so easy, Christine opens the door and asks, "Please are you through? Let's go to the movies."

W O R K O U T   3 3

Thighs still sore, so today I decide to do more *calves-abs-aerobics*. I turn to an ab-aerobic circuit arranging abdominal and aerobic exercises in the following order:

hanging knee ups
crunches
treadmill
leg raises
rowing
seated twist
stationary bike
one-arm cable crunches
  I do reps at each station for a minute before hopping to the next and resume without stopping reps continually for 20 minutes, going around the circuit twice.

After the workout, I appreciate this time-saving way to train abs and cardio at the same time. I call it ab-aerobics.

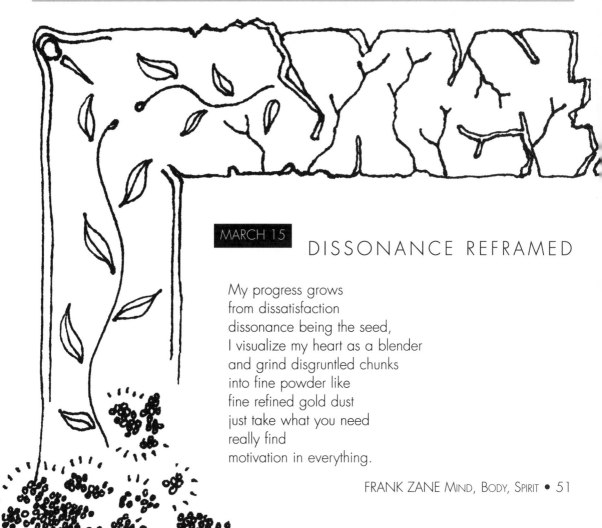

MARCH 15   DISSONANCE REFRAMED

My progress grows
from dissatisfaction
dissonance being the seed,
I visualize my heart as a blender
and grind disgruntled chunks
into fine powder like
fine refined gold dust
just take what you need
really find
motivation in everything.

W O R K O U T   3 4

Iwill do *chest-shoulder-triceps* workout today following the usual warm-ups:

70-degree incline dumbbell front press
  12 reps with 50 pounds, then 10 reps with 55 pounds,
  doing slow negatives; it takes a minute to do each of
  two sets, doing doorway stretch in between
low incline dumbbell press
  eight reps with 55 pounds, then six reps with 60
  pounds using the slowest negatives, over 10 seconds
pec deck
  115 pounds for 12 reps, 130 for 10, 145 for eight
dips
  13 reps, rested a minute, then 12
dumbbell pullover
  55 pounds for 10 reps, 60 for eight
triceps pressdown
  10 reps with 70 pounds, then nine with 80
rear deltoid dumbbell raises
  two sets of 10 reps with 25 pounds
one-arm dumbbell triceps extension
  12 reps with 25 pounds, then 10 with 30
one-arm dumbbell side raise
  12 reps with 20 pounds, then 10 with 25
rowing
  750 meters in four minutes

  ABS
knee up
crunches
one-arm cable crunch
  three sets of 30 reps each exercise

DINNER

Early dinner makes me thinner
so we're in our favorite fish restaurant at 5 P.M.
have broiled swordfish, tossed salad with oil and vinegar
small baked potato with steamed broccoli. Meal a delight
drinking coffee but no dessert.
I saw abs in the mirror that night.

WALKING MY DOG

Hit the road at sunrise with Tyler
on his leash, walk around the block
a couple times, we're both doing fine,
and walk the last hundred yards backwards
like a football linebacker but with
dog on a leash who guides me to the finish.
I notice how good my hamstrings, butt
and lower back feel after this.

ABS

Made an observation recently
that waistline, mine at least,
is a very dynamic area where
fat grows after a feast
and goes after a fast.
This storage site circles the middle
of the body all right, and ab work is needed
like 200 or 300 total reps three or four times a week
to make the waist tight.
Any of the ab routines I've given will do
but only if you watch how you eat.
Aerobics help too.

THE EARTH IS ME

From all I can see
the earth is just like my body
and the oceans too.
With each season that's new
a new trend is begun
that runs to completion.
Just as Winter's not Spring
get enough rest
overtraining is not the thing.

WINTER WORKOUT SUMMARY

DATE	MY WORKOUT	YOUR WORKOUT
Jan 1	full body	
Jan 3	full body	
Jan 5	upper body, abs	
Jan 8	legs, abs, aerobics	
Jan 10	back, biceps, forearms, abs	
Jan 13	legs, abs, aerobics	
Jan 15	chest, shoulders, triceps, abs, aerobics	
Jan 17	back, biceps, forearms, abs	
Jan 19	aerobics, legs, abs	
Jan 21	chest, shoulders, triceps, ab-aerobics	
Jan 22	abs, aerobics	
Jan 26	back	
Jan 27	back, biceps, forearms, abs	
Jan 30	legs, abs	
Feb 1	chest, shoulders, triceps, abs	
Feb 4	back, biceps, forearms, abs, aerobics	
Feb 6	legs, abs	
Feb 8	chest, shoulders, triceps, abs, aerobics	
Feb 11	back, biceps, forearms, abs	
Feb 13	legs, ab-aerobics	
Feb 15	chest, shoulders, triceps, abs, aerobics	
Feb 18	back, biceps, forearms, abs, aerobics	
Feb 19	legs, ab-aerobics	
Feb 21	chest, shoulders, triceps, abs, aerobics	
Feb 23	back, biceps, forearms, abs, aerobics	
Feb 26	legs, abs	
Feb 28	chest, shoulders, triceps, abs	
Mar 1	legs, abs	
Mar 4	abs, aerobics	

Mar 5	back, biceps, forearms, abs
Mar 6	legs, abs
Mar 8	chest, shoulders, triceps, abs, aerobics
Mar 11	back, biceps, forearms, ab-aerobics
Mar 13	thighs
Mar 14	calves, ab-aerobics
Mar 16	chest, shoulders, triceps, abs, aerobics
Mar 18	walking

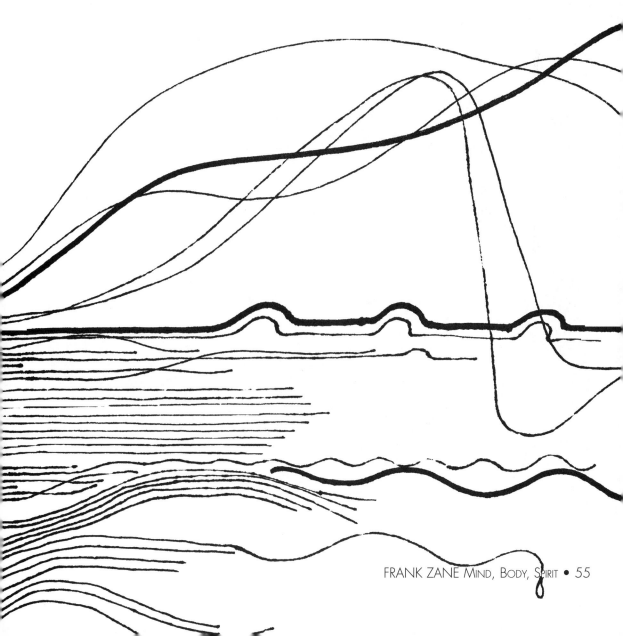

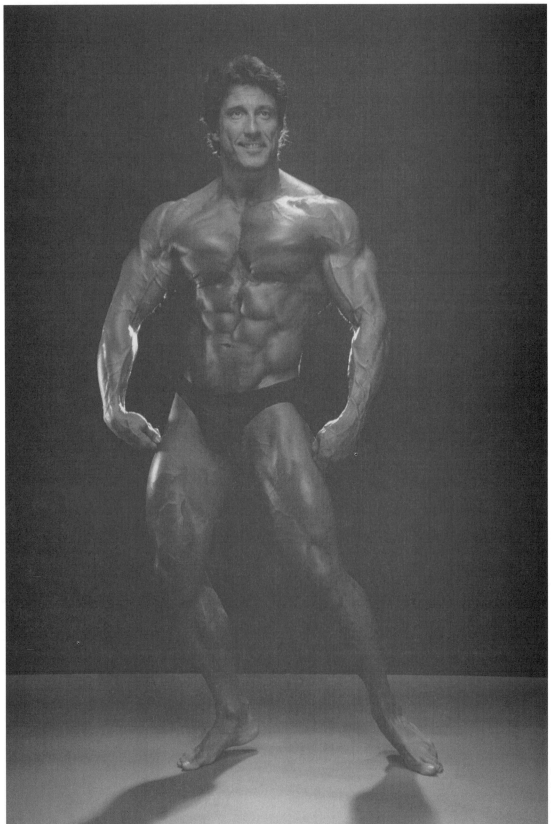

SPRING DIARY

Plants grow single mindedly
undisturbed by others
always fulfilling their wish
welcoming change
without hesitating
no abiding self to complain
about not making gains.
For plants know
when it's time to grow
then reach their peak
and finally blossom and bear fruit.
How I long for, how I seek
the plant's intuitivness
is quite unique.

W O R K O U T   3 5

Generally, doing more than four sets is unnecessary unless you are working each body part with only one exercise. So let's assume you're in a gym and you want to do one exercise for each bodypart. First, decide what exercises to perform, then limit your workout to no more than 30 total sets for upper body. You could even do seven exercises times four sets, increasing the weight for each set by five pounds while keeping your reps between eight and 12. Try this *upper body* routine:

**incline dumbbell bench press at 30 degrees
(for upper pecs)
front pulldown (for lats)
dumbbell pullover
interspersed with one-arm shoulder stretches**

TRICEPS AND DELTS
**one-arm dumbbell extension
one-arm dumbbell side raise**

BICEPS AND FOREARMS
curl dumbbells face down on steep incline bench
stopping a second at the top with slow slow negatives each rep
barbell wrist curl

hanging knee up or leg raises
no more than four sets of 30 reps

AM I ME OR NOT?

Jung says there's a self
Zen says there's not.
Think both are true
and you believe a lot.
Everything I think
becomes nothing
in the blink
of an eye
so I wink, why
I'm on the brink
of deep enlightened glory
but don't worry
that's only half the story
closing my eyes I sink
into a blurry Satori.

WORKOUT 36

Today I do *legs* with one set of *thigh* and *calf* exercises combined with two minutes on aerobic devices in between:

leg extension
leg curl
erect squat
    all for 10 reps, followed by two minutes on stationary bike
leg press
hip machine
standing one-legged curl
    all for 10 reps, treadmill for two minutes
standing calf raises
leg press
donkeys
seated calf raises
    all for 15 reps, followed by two minutes of walking around
hanging knee ups
crunches
seated twist
    all for 30 reps, followed by a three-minute rest before going around my circuit once more

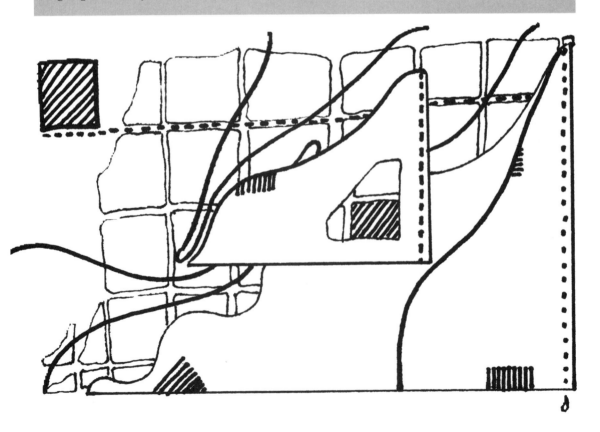

BODHIBUILDING

Science is now entertaining what ancient schools
of wisdom have known for thousands of years:
Interpenetrating the physical body we inhabit are
resonant systems which when entrained on a regular basis
develop into a form, a higher coherent being.
Building this body is called Bodhibuilding
whose goal is awakening the inherent enlightened nature in all of us.
Included is the bodybuilding of weights, sets, reps, protein,
fat, carbohydrate, rest, competition, attitude.
Bodhibuilding seeks not only to develop the physical muscular body,
but also the awakened Bodhi body, the next step in human evolution.
This body of consciousness is also called soul
enlightened, subtle, etheric, astral, dream body our goal
self-image, body of music, body of light, Sambodhi
known as Sambhogakaya, body of wisdom, compassion
enjoyment, self-realization, energy body.
True nature means more than flesh and bones
it's as if my body sings with new energy past winter.
Now lavender rosebuds open
while Bermuda grass turns green
I can smell white orange blossoms
as birds sing atop eucalyptus trees
good-bye death of winter
hello birth of spring
bringing progress
everywhere
in everything.

WORKOUT 37

A trip by car or plane is a workout out in itself. Planning one tomorrow, I decide not to weight train and instead do *stretching*—holding each stretch 20 seconds without bounce—followed by *aerobics*:

two-arm lat stretch
doorway stretch
one-arm lat stretch
one-arm shoulder stretch
arms back stretch
one-arm rear delt stretch
two-arm lat stretch
one leg up stretch
one leg back stretch
calf stretch

ABS
leg raise
crunches
seated twist
two sets of 30 reps each

ARIZONA GEM EXPEDITION

Speeding east on I-10
alongside the road
dense scattered palm trees
silhouette in the mist
against the hills
of La Quinta
and Indian Wells
in the distance
extending beyond the rim
of Coachella Valley.
Mountains of Indio
flat stratified rock
looked like ice covered with snow
just past 29 Palms exit
on my right saw a rainbow
whose bent vertical bow shot
mighty arrows of sunlight
right through morning sky already hot.

My, I watched wispy green
rows of creosote trees
trace a crooked line
across bright yellow sand
and mud-colored towers
where telephone poles stand
like toothpicks parallel
for miles and miles
across the vanishing land
where there's only 16 more miles
left to Blythe, then appear
jagged mountain castles
like a Camelot
due south of Quartzite.
In this dusty tent city
we find pretty gemstones for Christine
for me a blow gun
and bowie knife.

MEDITATE THEN WORKOUT 38

While there are many ways to meditate, I've found that shooting my new blowgun an interesting variation to improve my focus. First, I get up and meditate, then while in a relaxed state I shoot darts at a target until one hits the center. When three are centered, I make breakfast, eat, work a bit, write, read, then go to the gym and begin an intensive *chest-shoulder-triceps* workout after first doing doorway stretching.

lightweight barbell presses on 30-degree incline
15 reps, four-second negatives, then 10 reps with 140 pounds, then more doorway stretching

dumbbell press on 70-degree incline
10 reps with 45 and 50 pounds

peck deck
10 reps with 130 and 145 pounds

dip machine
10 reps with 150 and 160 pounds

dumbbell pullover
two sets of 10 reps with 80 pounds

{ **rear delt machine**
two sets of 10 reps with 100 pounds
pressdown
two sets of 10 reps with 70 pounds

{ **one-arm dumbbell extension**
two sets of 10 reps with 30 pounds
one-arm dumbbell side raises
two sets of 10 reps with 20 pounds

{ **knee up**
partial situp
one-arm cable crunch
two sets of 30 reps each
rowed
1000 meters in five minutes

LAST NIGHT

Head upstairs
before going to bed and
tripped oh, feigned
a heavy entrance into bed
and instead
ate my date
brushed my teeth
then fell asleep
make no mistake
six hours deep sleep
relaxed deep, deeper down inside.
Then dream, wondering
what motivates me to keep inspired.
Early morning, get up, take a leak
I'm so tired I go back to sleep.
Remembering back
re-dream a 1970s familiar theme
where only two characters, actors deemed
Diana Bowl and Louie
Prima bowl on
TV, both of whom
worked as a team.
Known for miles around
as the best bowlers in town,
Primo drove 100 miles a week
combining 15 milly Gramola bars daily from Diana
not worried about getting fat, you cannot
not on that in those days.
But that was then, this is now
a growing cast of actors shove, share center stage
all playing the same part at the same time
I awoke amazed, wondering how
this ridiculous play isn't dying by now.

MY FATHER

Tired today, worked instead, then lying around after
eating almost a pound of turkey and
a lettuce, apple, walnut, cheese salad
found myself thinking of my father
the electrician, father, husband
radio and TV technician
could fix anything broken
and he fixed everything
our house at 11 Franklin Street wired with his own hands
and a little bit with mine
on a hill in Pennsylvania to this day it still stands
worked hard to pay all the bills
put food on the table for my mother, brother, and me
two jobs, by day and weekends revived dead TVs
electrician by night for number 5 Loree Colliery
I still remember the ominous black brooding coal breakers
monstrous dark dank buildings
with tunnels declining 45 degrees, down
for hundreds of feet before they stopped
coal cars elevated 50-pound coal rocks all the way to the top
coal boulders roll tumbling deep down the decline and stop
at the bottom broken into much smaller pieces.
After school and weekends I saw miners
like my Uncle Johnny coming up from the mines
hard helmeted black faces and hands
coal dust all over everywhere
even in their lungs.
Never did I ever see my father this way
maybe, except once, on a hunch, I went to Loree
saw my father running around, face dirty
but the last time I visited there he was sitting
with his feet up on a desk drinking a quart of milk
told me he only worked when things broke.
The miners were all friends
my father's pal Paul Thomas
owned a bar in Larksville and especially
had a huge right biceps
which beat everyone in arm wrestling.

WORKOUT 39
— ATTAINMENT BEGINNING

I'm able to get into a single-minded concentration, a state the yogis call Samadhi. Before the 1979 Mr. Olympia contest, I was able to sustain that concentration for weeks at a time. But now it doesn't last. So, I must focus on one thing at a time and forget everything else. With the vision of Paul Thomas' biceps in my mind, I work on *back-biceps-forearms* remembering to pull hard on all movements, while being careful not to superset two pulling exercises in a row.

{ **pulldown**
155 pounds for 12 reps, 170 for 10
cable crossover behind neck
two sets of 20 reps with 40 pounds (the best combination for upper lats I know)

{ **low cable row**
10 reps at 150 and 165 pounds
dumbbell shrug
two sets of 20 reps with 65 pounds

one-arm cable rowing
two sets of 10 reps at 100 pounds, one-arm lat stretch after each set

dumbbell concentration curls
nonstop sets of 12, 10, and eight reps with 30 pounds each arm

curling face down on incline bench
two arms for two sets of 10 reps with 30-pound dumbbells

preacher bench
12 and 10 reps at 80 and 90 pounds

{ **reverse wrist curl**
two sets of 12 reps
wrist curl
two sets of 12 reps
gripper
two sets of 12 reps

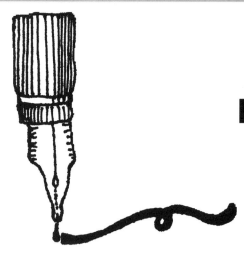

DREAMING INK

Dreaming toward morning
ink told behavior
these are my words
write them down now
savor them afterwards.

WORKOUT 40

Because legs wear out first in the aged, I always plan my sessions to avoid any kind of leg injury. With ab work, it is unnecessary to do too many total reps at this stage. I used to do one thousand a day. It sure paid off in great abs but my lower back usually was sore and sometimes still hurts today. Now do 1000 abs reps—*not* a day—but a week, along with aerobics for one to two hours a week. I seek the best nutrition all the time keeping my fat calories under 25 percent and protein at least one gram per pound of bodyweight with carbs a little higher than protein intake. I eat starches early in the day. This gives me enough energy to work out and make gains.

leg extension
leg curl
   both: 15, 12, and 10 reps increasing the weight 10 pounds each set, and one minute rest between sets
squatting
   (with upper body erect)
   15, 12, and 10 reps increasing the weight 10 pounds each set, and one minute rest between sets
rest three minutes
standing calf raises
   15 reps, holding five seconds at the top
leg press calf raise
   15 reps, holding five seconds at the top
donkeys
   15 reps, holding five seconds at the top
seated calf raises
   15 reps, holding five seconds at the top
treadmill
   11 minutes at 3.3 miles per hour followed by some ab work

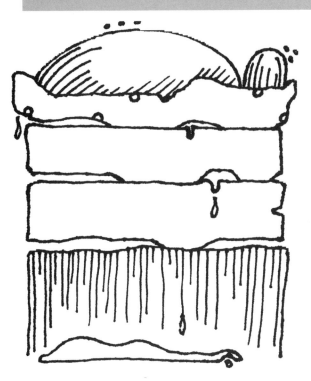

INEVITABLE ACCEPTANCE OF AGE

"Accept old age
and death, realize
it's just as wise
at this stage
to have a good death
as to have a good life
aim in either no strife."
So said the wife
in my dream of a sage.

FRANK ZANE MIND, BODY, SPIRIT • 67

WORKOUT 41

I'm doing a *chest-shoulder-tricep* workout today with a client.

one-arm shoulder stretch
70-degree dumbbell front press
40 pounds for 15 reps, 45 for 12

UPPER PECS
30-degree dumbbell press
two sets of 15 reps with 45 pounds, then 12 reps with
50 pounds, stretching deep down when the dumbbells reach the bottom of each rep and not locking
out at the top, holding tension all through the set
pec deck
115 pounds for 15 reps, 130 for 12
dip
two sets of 10 reps with bodyweight
close-grip barbell bench press
two sets of 10 reps with 100 pounds, doing very slow
negatives
bent over dumbbell raises
two sets of 12 reps with 20-pound dumbbells for rear
delts
{ **one-arm dumbbell extension**
one-arm side cable raises
two sets of 10 reps with 30 pounds on each
rowing
1000 meters

ABS
partial situp
one-arm cable crunch
leg raises
three sets of 30 reps

CORN GROWING

Driving to San Diego today saw
away in the field
stand row upon row
stalks of corn
masters of form
being reborn
green growing

ears of concern
wearing away
like loose bales of hay
from strong gusts of wind
blowing all day
away in the field.

W O R K O U T   4 2

Today it is time to work on *back-biceps-forearms*. For the sake of the elbows, pulling exercises are best done with a palms parallel grip. I do all my pulldowns and rows this way because it gives me a pump and keeps my elbows injury free

front pulldown
  10 reps with 150, 160, and 170 pounds, not locking out and pulling all the way down to my upper chest
low cable row
  10 reps with 140 and 150 pounds
one-arm dumbbell row
  two sets of 10 reps with 70 pounds, with one-arm lat stretch between sets
close parallel grip pulldown
  two sets of 12 reps with 140 pounds
60-pound dumbbell shrugs
  two sets of 20 reps

  BICEPS
alternate dumbbell curl
  12 reps with 35 pounds, 10 with 40
dumbbell concentration curl
  two sets of 10 rep with 30 pounds

  FOREARMS
barbell reverse curl
  two sets of 10 reps with 70 pounds
barbell wrist curl
  two sets of 20 reps with 90 pounds

  ABS
leg raise
partial situp
one-arm cable crunches
  three sets of 30 reps each

THE MIDDLE WAY

The Middle Way:
means going all the way
right down the middle.
Not half way
commitment always needed
it's mean, mode, median
measuring central tendency
in all situations
doing just enough
nothing's exceeded
gets more from less
parsimony, elegance
have to say
it's not for extremists
avoids losing your way
today goes straight
to the source of course
stays away
from nay sayers.
This railroad train
with parallel tracks
right down the middle
of the plain, runs everyday
goal straight ahead
services this way
enjoy the scenery, foray
take the "En" train
it's bound to pay
way off in the end
and along the way
total equilibrium
through focused concentration
knowing everything under the sun
working, growing, getting things done.

WORKOUT 43

Thighs have always been my strongest body part. I could squat with 300 pounds for sets of 10 when I was 18. I've found the only time I need to squat heavier is when I want to gain a few pounds. Caution: heavy squatting can wreck your lower back and knees. This routine makes more sense:

leg extension
Leg Blaster squat
   two sets of 10 reps each
leg curl
leg press
   two sets of 10 reps each, followed by a three minutes rest

   CALVES
standing calf raises
   two sets of 15 reps, holding five seconds at the top of each
donkeys
   two sets of 15 reps, holding five seconds at the top of each
seated calf raises
   two sets of 15 reps, holding five seconds at the top of each

leg raises
crunches
   two sets of 30 reps each
stationary bike
   10 minutes
treadmill
   10 minutes

DEFINITELY DEFINITION

Spring time a new rendition, renew training structure inspiration
without waiting or inhibition now find clear definition.
Webster's definition means a creation
distinct definite being sharp outline giving
specific statement of meaning always pursuing more definition
might call my life a search for the meaning of things
Two sides this coin called definition
one is body regimental, the other is existential.
First is training technology, physiology, stretching, exercise
food supplements, drugs, stress, sleep, sun, therapy.
Existential side feeling, appreciation, intuition, love, mind, heart, spirit.
One is science, structure, mathematics—other is art, inspiration, poetry
together form the meaning of things.
This is definitely definition.

WORKOUT 44

Chest-shoulder-triceps workout gives the best pump of all through working the pushing, lateral raising, and the extending muscles.

30-degree dumbbell press
  10 reps with 50 and 55 pounds
pec deck
  10 reps with 115 and 130 pounds
dumbbell pullover
  12 reps with 50 pounds and 10 reps with 55 pounds
dip
  two sets of 10 reps with bodyweight
one-arm tricep extension
  10 reps at 30 pounds, eight at 35
one-arm side raise one-arm with dumb-bell
  10 reps at 15 pounds, eight at 20

300 total reps of the usual abdominal stuff
treadmill
  20 minutes

SCULPTURE

Bodhibuilding sculptor creates a statue not of clay
because both sculptor and statue are the same
layer upon layer form
muscle size and proportion
aesthetic symmetrical lines
nothing's too big, small, loose, or tight
composition perfect, everything's just right
this kind of development takes a lifetime
to build definition
maximize muscle size.
First build some size so there's something to define
but not so fast that muscle expands out of your skin
say no to stretch marks and as fast as you please
gradually grow more proportionate muscles, you'll be glad you did
no one muscle group overshadows any other
in a perfect body all muscles are brothers
all bodyparts proportionally shout
as every single muscle stands out.

WORKOUT 45

This is a ***back-biceps-forearms*** workout I did years ago but with weights I'd use today:

LATS

one-arm dumbbell row
10 reps with 60, 65, and 70 pounds, each set followed with one-arm lat stretch

wide grip pulldown behind the neck
150 and 160 pounds for 10 reps, although I don't do this exercise anymore because it hurts my shoulder

T-bar row
(simply an Olympic bar stuck in a corner with 70 pounds loaded on one end) three sets of 10 reps adding 10 pounds each set

BICEPS

alternate dumbbell curl
35 pounds for 12 reps, 40 for 10, and 45 for eight

one-arm dumbbell concentration curl
10 reps with each arm using 30 pounds nonstop with slow negatives

reverse curl
three sets of 10 reps with 85 pounds

crunches
hanging knee ups
seated twist
three tri-sets of 30 reps each

rowing
500 meters

TEAM DREAM THEME

Had a dream
I was on a team
of some kind
as an observer
in a school
all dressed up fine
skirts, coats, and ties
don't remember many women there
mostly only guys
I was sitting there
in assembly
ready to be recognized
as one of the team
but toward the end
everyone had been called on stage
but me
so I left, unrecognized
now I'm wise
as I think of this dream
I feel unrecognized, uncompromised but
motivated
and appreciate why I've never been
a member of this team
seems I can do things better myself
self-reliance has always been my theme
when I want something done right
I do it myself
or ask Christine.

WORKOUT 46

Legs have always been an easy body part for me, so today I concentrate on aerobics instead of the usual leg training spree:

treadmill
 20 minutes, from -2 up to 12 degrees
stationary bike
 20 minutes

GOALS

Making continuous progress to the full
needs a plan to reach predetermined goals
coming in two varieties:
a short term goal you reach in 13 weeks
the length of a season, you seek
to develop a trend, start to get in shape
so you arrive where you want to be and beyond
at the end of each training season.
Know that Nature always reaches her goal
a new trend in the beginning
finishing it at the season's end.
Long term goal's for the entire year
the sum of the goals you reach
each season, brings you near
best possible body you can seek
improvement destination
stretching 52 weeks.

WORKOUT 47

Training the *chest-shoulders-triceps* requires cutting down on rest between sets to give maximum definition and stamina. The following half-hour workout is organized in tri-sets as a way to optimize pump and muscular striations.

{ **front press**
pec deck
pullover
   two sets of 10 reps each

{ **30-degree incline barbell press**
rear delt machine
dip machine
   two sets of 10 reps each

{ **one-arm dumbbell triceps extension**
one-arm dumbbell side raise
   two sets of 10 reps each

EATEN UP

In a dream I call "the hungry jungle"
a man kills a wild cat
my cat kills a yellow bird
before that, the bird ate a worm
originally the worm ate the soil.
In life's hierarchy of survival fittest
higher life devours
everything underneath toils
sacrificial dying, overpowered
food chain of pain.
Is dying a karmic reprimand?
Does killing even the score?
Is the wheel turning
life force cruel
or just indifferent?

WORKOUT 48

Today I train *back-biceps-forearms*.

front pulldown
   12, 10, and eight reps with 160, 170, and 180 pounds
low cable row
   10 reps with 150 and 160 pounds
one-arm cable row
   two sets of 12 reps with 100 pounds each arm
dumbbell shrugs
   two sets of 20 reps with 65-pounders
one-arm concentration dumbbell curl
   30 pounds of two nonstop sets of 10 reps
face down incline alternate dumbbell curl
   12 reps with 30 pounds, 10 reps with 35, eight reps
   with 40
reverse wrist curl
   two sets of 10 reps with 50 pounds
barbell wrist curl
   two sets of 15 reps with 75 pounds

   ABS
crunches
   three sets of 30 reps
leg raises
   three sets of 30 reps
seated twist
   three sets of 40 reps

MY CATS

Randolph, Carey, Tyrone, Tim
and Zorro, cat of the year
wherever I am he's always near
every morning sits atop my lap
purring, lots of fur
all over the place.
Four cats compete for my lap everyday
in their own unique time and way
Zorrow each morrow
Randolph anytime
day or night
Carey's on Christine's lap at breakfast
Timmy jumps up on me
two or three times every night
sometimes there's a fight
under the bed between
Timmy and Tyrone
24-pound Jabba the Hutt this fat cat wide
moans at the back porch door
each morning when he's not inside
yellow eyed gray balloon boy
Timmy thinks of him as a big toy
lies with his head
resting on bowl of water
sneaks up to be petted
when sitting on the toilet
boy, let any of them stay
inside all the time and
I would need more than two hands.

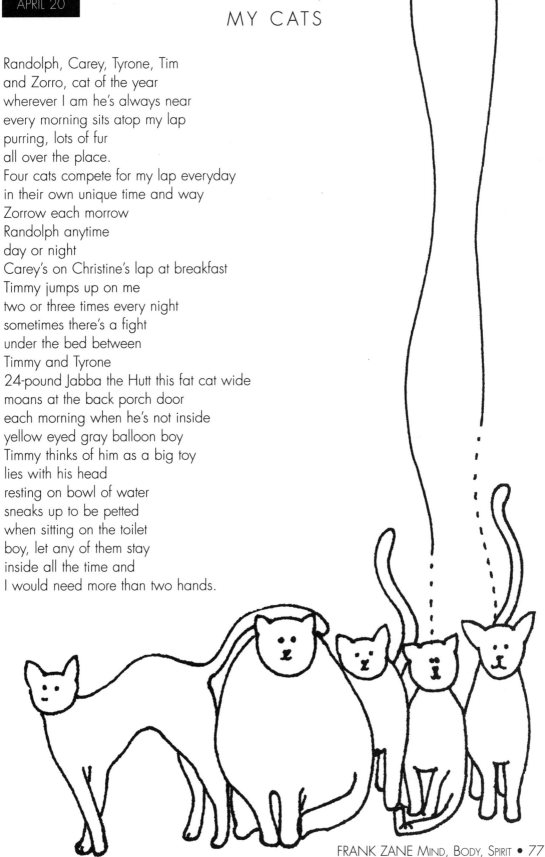

A GREAT LATE LUNCH

Decided to take a day off from working out today
and after an early morning half hour walk with my dog Tyler
(walked 200 yard backwards) ate a light breakfast:
amino acids, an orange, liver extract, germ oil concentrate
multiple vitamin-minerals, a slice of whole grain toast
with a teaspoon of dark sesame oil soaked in
and a cup of peppermint tea.
Good oils kill hunger and I didn't eat again until 11 A.M.
when I had three slices of low fat ham with a small baked yam
and the same supplements as breakfast.
Not hungry again until 5 P.M. when I ate a three-egg-spinach-swiss-cheese omelet.
Before bed had amino acids and a large Rome apple.

WORKOUT 49

A question I'm often asked about training is, "What are you thinking about when doing a set?" The answer is *counting*: keeping track of reps and attending to the pump I get. The most frequently used numbers are 1, 2, 3, 4, 6, 8, 9, 10, 11, 12, 13, 14, 15, 18, 20, 25, 30, 40, 50, and 100. Using them helps me get a great pump and increase my workout intensity. Today is a *leg* workout, pretty much the same workout with the same reps and weights as last time:

leg extension
two sets of 10 reps
leg curl
two sets of 10 reps
Leg Blaster squat
two sets of 10 reps
leg press
two sets of 10 reps
hip machine
two sets of 10 reps
standing one leg curl
two sets of 10 reps

CALVES
standing calf raise
one set of 15 reps holding five seconds at the top
seated calf raise
one set of 15 reps holding five seconds at the top
donkey calf raise
one set of 15 reps holding five seconds at the top
calf raises on leg press machine
one set of 15 reps holding five seconds at the top

ABS (300 total reps)
hanging knee ups
crunches
one-arm cable crunches

CENTERED, ON TARGET

Best blowgun morning yet
many darts right in the center
those that aren't, I pull out
and shoot over, and over
until they're closer together
a tight group
none far apart from each other.

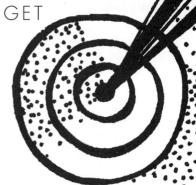

WORKOUT 50

After hours of searching, I uncovered my training journals. Twenty-one hand-written books covering training sessions from 1959, 1968, 1974-1986, 1990 to the present. The years my training was serious enough to get in great shape, I recorded not only the workouts with numbers of sets, reps, and pounds, but also contest posing routines, foods I ate, supplements I took, and dreams I had. So first a *chest-shoulder-triceps* workout from spring 1994:

30-degree incline barbell press
120 pounds for 10 reps, 130 for eight, 140 for six using a 10-second negative

70-degree incline dumbbell press
45 pounds for 10 reps, 50 for seven, deep stretch at the bottom and slow negatives

pec deck
115 pounds for 12 reps, 130 for 10

cable crossover
40 pounds for two sets of 10 reps

parallel dips
two sets of 10 reps

dumbbell pullover
12 reps with 60 pounds, and 10 with 65

rear deltoid bent over dumbbell raises
two sets of 12 with 25 pounds

triceps pressdown
12 reps with 70 pounds and 10 with 75

one-arm dumbbell extension
32.5 pounds for 10 reps and 35 for eight

one-arm dumbbell side raises
15 and 17.5 pounds both for 12 reps with one arm

two-arm tricep cable extension
two sets of 12 reps with 50 pounds

dumbbell pronated side raises
two sets of 12 reps with 17.5 pounds

ABS
crunches
two sets of 50 reps

leg raises
two sets of 30 reps

seated twist
two sets of 100 reps

ODE TO ABS BONSAI

Read where I go to Tokyo in the mid-70s
as a guest at Mr. Japan
where little bonsai physiques
with abs planted deep in the sand
160 glistening pip-squeaks on stage
small acorn head man
growing beautiful trees
squeezed into plan
little bonsai physique
like abs

send little acorn helmeted men
to do battle
in the middle
of your body
victorious at attention
rows and columns
linea alba down the middle
little bonsai physique
like abs.

BIRTH AND YOUTH

My uncle Frank was killed riding his bike
right before I was born and as I grew up
everyone said, "You're just like your Uncle Frank"
so I thought I was him, I identified
was named after him
and everything he liked to do
I did too, like hiking in the woods
Buttermilk Falls always felt so familiar
went there almost every Saturday early in the morning
knapsack, canteen of water
three eggs in a jar kept cold in a stream
cooked bacon frying in my pan
breakfast never tasted so good
would hike all day, laze, gaze at the waterfall
and forest of trees
contemplating nature
of spring, summer, fallen autumn leaves
time flew quickly and soon
hike two miles home in late afternoon.

WORKOUT 51

Back in 1991 here was my *back-biceps-forearms* workout the day after my 49th birthday:

front pulldown
160 and 170 pounds for 10 reps
crossover behind neck
40 and 50 pounds for 12 reps
low cable row
150 and 160 pounds for 10 reps
bent over rear cable raise
two sets of 10 reps with 20 pounds
close grip pulldown
12 reps with 140, 10 with 150
reverse pec deck
two sets of 12 reps with 65 pounds
one-arm cable row
two sets with 100 pounds each arm, and one-arm lat
stretch after each set

BICEPS
one-arm seated curl
30 pounds for 12 reps and 35 pounds for 10 reps
face down incline dumbbell curl
two sets of 10 reps with 25 pounds
preacher cable curl
two sets of 12 reps with 80 pounds

FOREARMS
barbell reverse curl
two sets with 65 pounds for 10 reps
barbell wrist curl
two sets with 65 pounds for 20 reps
gripper
two sets for 20 reps
rowing
1000 meters in a little over six minutes

THIS MORNING AT 6 A.M.

Listening to Bach's Brandenburg Concerto number three
kept up with some of the tune blowing and drawing deep on my
Hohner Super 16-hole Chromonica 64
bought in Tijuana Mexico back in 1973 for 20 dollars,
today it costs 10 times more.
I played spontaneously a "Blow Draw Sliding Scale Tune in the Key of C"
then using my sharps and flats button pushing single and multiple variationally
different tempos according to my feeling and my breathing.
Now notes of tune go round in my head instead of radio or TV.
Kerouac's List of Essentials says "Something you feel will find its own form . . .
Blow as deep as you want to blow"
as I continue to practice my own
ascending descending draw blow harmonica concerto.

WORKOUT 52

Because of a sore lower back, I do this *thighs-calves-abs* workout in order to maximize calves, quads and hamstrings while taking it easy on the lower back and knees:

sissy squat with Leg Blaster
  three sets of 20 reps, keeping tension on thighs
  throughout the movement
standing calf raise with Leg Blaster
  three sets of 20 reps
incline leg raise
  three sets of 30 reps

This is a lower body-ab workout with three exercises

HARMONICA SYMPONEA

Played my harmonica
four octave 16 hole
chromonica 64
this morning
half hour or more
blow draw symposia
musical breath
inspires my high
look at the wall
trees shoot way up out the window
and on wall photographs
stand among beaming trees
above painted heart with wings
glance ascending, noticing
how tall they grow up these
wagon wheel and yucca plant photos in black and white
same radial symmetry
wheels of life
many spokes radiate the from center
your chief feature says Gurdjieff.
Really eight spokes are all you need
to connect rim with center
Christine's photographs
help me understand it better.

WORKOUT 53

From my June 27, 1991, diary entry, I find this *chest-shoulder-triceps* workout

70-degree incline dumbbell front press
  12 reps with 40 pounds, 10 with 45, eight with 50
pec deck
  130 pounds for 12 reps, 145 for 10
dip machine
  160 and 170 pounds for 10 reps
cable crossover
  10 reps with 50 then 60 pounds
dumbbell pullover
  two sets of 10 reps with 65 pounds
stiff arm pulldown
  two sets of 10 reps with 60 pounds
  with doorway stretch between each set
pressdown
  10 reps with 70 and 80 pounds
bent over dumbbell rear delt raises
  two sets of 12 reps with 25 pounds

{ **dumbbell kickbacks**
pronated side dumbbell raise
  two sets of 12 reps with 25 pounds for each
one-arm dumbbell extension
  two sets with 35 pounds for 10 reps
dumbbell side raise
  two sets with 25 pounds for 10 reps
rowing
  1000 meters in just under six minutes

abs exercises
  320 total reps

I rode my bike one mile round trip to the post office, but was glad I was finished when I got home.

EXISTENCE

Now as I write a beautiful sunrise
in the eastern sky stratifies the horizon
into layers of pink purple blue
sinking deep into mind innermost
asking, "If I weren't here right now
would this sunrise exist?"

and "If I didn't record that workout
in my diary would it exist too?"
The night's dream answer was a clear
  voice
that said "all that exists is in your mind.
Does that surprise you?"

THE PULSE OF WORKOUT 54

After my 44th birthday in 1986, I discovered in my diaries that I used to check my pulse after each set.

{ **partial situp**
pulley knee in
  four sets of 30 reps

one-arm cable crunch
  two nonstop sets each arm holding 75 pounds

seated twists
  50 reps

hyperextensions
  20 reps (my pulse was 127 after this ab work)

low cable row
  two sets of 20 reps with 160 pounds (my pulse went to 165 beats per minute)

deadlift from knees up
  (with a wide grip)
  20 reps and 235 pounds (my pulse hovered around 156)

front pulldown
  after the third set of 20 reps with 160 pounds, my pulse still at 154

one-arm cable row
  20 reps with 75 pounds each arm (my pulse was 153)

preacher cable curl
  two sets of 10 reps with 70 pounds

seated 30-pound dumbbell curls
  two sets of 12 reps (my pulse dropped to 148)

{ **barbell reverse curl**
wrist curl
  two sets each of 10 reps with 60 pounds (my pulse was 142)

stationary bike
  four miles in 12 minutes at 90 revolutions a minute (ended my workout with pulse at 130—right on target)

INNUMERABLE VARIATIONS
OF WORKOUTS AND WORDS

Like an infant knowing only 10 words
suppose composing sentences using only these.
How many sentences could an infant compose with 10 words?
Barring meaning arranging 10 words in all possible orders
three million six hundred twenty eight thousand eight hundred
different sentences are possible with a vocabulary of 10 words.
Yet infant also has access to 9-word, 8-, 7-, 6-, 5-, 4-, 3-, 2-, 1-word sentences, too
adding up to four million thirty seven thousand nine hundred thirteen
so you can see even with a vocabulary
limited to only 10 what can be
imagine what you can do with access
in excess of 10,000 words or more
so much we can say in so many ways
we'll never say it
and in a similar way
there's lots of different workouts
we can do as we expand our vocabulary of exercises.
A beginner must first master about 10 exercises
plus a few stretches.
Then as muscles grow
perfect even more,
do as many different exercises as you can do in good form
expanding workout repertoire
you'll never run out of different workout routines
which are not even routine anymore you can bet
everything works when you let it.
Get it?
Expand, expanding word and exercise vocabulary
never running out of things to say, workouts to do
never any boredom becomes a guarantee.

LEG PULSATION WORKOUT 55

Looking back to first day of summer in 1986, I did this *leg-abs* workout while keeping track of my pulse.

leg extension
   three sets of 15 reps with 160 pounds (my pulse was 146)
Leg Blaster squat
   three sets of 20 reps with 135 pounds (pulse 163)
{**lunges on Leg Blaster**
   12 reps with 35 pounds, 10 with 40
leg curl
   20 with 70 pounds, 16 with 80 (pulse at 148 and 145 after each superset, respectively)
three minutes rest
standing calf raise
   two sets of 15 reps
seated calf raise
   two sets of 15 reps
donkeys
   two sets of 15 reps (pulse at 135)
ab-aerobics
   10 minutes
stationary bike
   10 minutes at 90 rpm (pulse staying right around 125 the whole time)

ESCAPE FROM MEXICO
RECURRING DREAM THEME

Dreaming I'm in Mexico and decide to get shoulder operation
give $125 deposit on surgery then change my mind and want to leave
after realizing how dumb this is check airline reservation
still four days left, got to hang around, buy gemstones get pesos in change
Looking at newspaper there's photos of Arnold and me on Ferris wheel
flexing muscles he does right biceps poses
while I flex my left triceps informally
suddenly find I'm home in Palm Springs, drove here I think
walking around my large yard at night looking for Christine
see her in upstairs bedroom over the gym, I want to
drink tea I bought in Mexico but don't
wake up instead realizing
escape from Mexico and other dream scenes recurring theme since 1976 in
   Mexico City
posing exhibition with Arnold and Franco Colombu.
Later had to pay Arnold for a dinner bill we still owed.
Who ever thought going there would be a vacation?
Secret safe in Mexico until a moment ago.

WORKOUT 56

Early on June 13, 1986, I went for a 20-minute bike ride in the Palm Springs foothills on my red steed, Fassi 12-speed. My pulse rose from 68 at the start, peaked at 170 while going 25 miles an hour in sixth gear, and returned to 68 at the end of seven miles after a five-minute rest. In the gym, I concentrated on *chest-shoulders-triceps*.

ABS
{ **partial situp**
  incline leg raise
  75 pound one-arm cable crunch
  three sets of 30 reps each
hyperextensions
two sets of 20 reps(pulse at 109)

CHEST
{ **45-degree incline dumbbell press**
  50 and 60 pounds for 10 reps
  V bar dips
  two sets of 10 reps with bodyweight (pulse at 153)
{ **40-pound cable crossover**
  60-pound dumbbell pullover
  two sets of 10 reps (pulse still at 153)

TRICEPS
one-arm dumbbell extension
two sets of eight reps with 30 pounds (pulse at 153)
70-pound pressdown
10 reps
25-pound dumbbell kickback
two sets of 10 reps (pulse down to 147 and my triceps were burning)

SHOULDERS
one-arm side cable raise
two nonstop sets of 10 reps with 30 pounds (pulse back to 153)
rear delt cable raise
two sets of 10 reps with 20 pounds
side dumbbell raise
two sets of 10 reps with 25 pounds (pulse around 150)

SPRING SALAD

Find myself eating more salads as warm weather approaches.
Today filled a large bowl with a head of Romaine lettuce,
mixed in eight ounces chicken, diced apple, four ounces swiss cheese,
handful of walnuts, chopped celery stalk, tablespoon walnut oil,
apple cider vinegar, tossed around, and ate it slowly
with rye crisp cracker and iced peppermint tea.

WORKOUT 57

In July 1985 I trained on a four-way split routine: Day One back-rear delts-abs; Day Two, calves-thighs-abs; Day Three, rest; Day Four, chest-delts-front and side; Day Five, biceps-triceps-forearms-abs; Day Six, rest or bicycle riding. This Day One workout includes *back-rear delts-abs*:

BACK

front pulldown
160 pounds for 12 reps, 170 for 11, 180 for 10 (my negatives are slower now than they were then)

low cable row
10 reps at 160, 170, and 180 pounds

T-bar row
100 pounds for 10 reps, 120 pounds for 10, 130 pounds for eight

one-arm dumbbell row
10 reps at 80, 85, and 90 pounds

REAR DELTS

bent over rear cable raise
three sets of 10 reps with 20 pounds

dumbbell shrug
three sets of 10 reps with 75 pounds

lightweight barbell press behind neck
three sets of 10 reps

pulldown behind neck
three sets 10 reps with 170 pounds

one-arm side cable raise
nonstop three sets of 10 reps with 20 pounds

ABS

{ **pulley knee**
three sets of 30 reps with 40 pounds
incline leg raise
crunches
three sets of 30 reps }

seated twists
80 reps

W O R K O U T   5 8

Day Two of the four-way split concentrates on *calves-thighs-abs*:

ABS

{ **incline leg raise**
crunches
three sets of 30 reps
seated twists
100 reps
hyperextension
two sets of 20 reps

one minute of rest

CALVES
donkey calf raise
200, 220, and 240 pounds for 20 reps
seated calf raise
80 and 90 pounds for 20 reps, then 100 pounds for 15 reps

THIGHS
leg curl
80 pounds for 12 reps, 90 for 11, 100 for 10
leg extension
160 pounds for 12 reps, 170 and 180 pounds for 11 reps
Leg Blaster squats
85 pounds for 16 reps, 135 for 12, 165 for 10
lunges
three sets of 10 reps with 40 pounds
stationary bike
15 minutes

DREAM HIGH

Before falling asleep, lying in bed thinking
Living is all we know
can't realize what dying's like
because haven't been dead yet
only dead tired
bend opposite course
after being wired
divorce mind thought
relax deep, expire . . . inspire . . .
and exhaling . . . as I inhale new life
expire deep . . . falling asleep
inhaling deep deeper down
holding on to breath of life longer and longer
exhaling all the way out more and more complete
inhaling think "I am one with desire"
dream of climbing high up ladder into the sky
my father and I climb higher and higher and reach the moon
then he shows me how to get back down
to earth with a back flip over and over
turning around and around down deep through clouds we land in
Cheyenne, Wyoming.

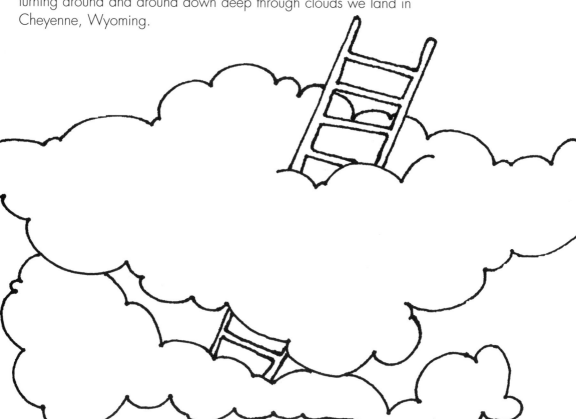

WORKOUT 59

I write in my diary that owning my body implies taking care to completely control my workout and nutrition. On July 19, 1985, in my Palm Springs gym, I begin Day Four of the four-way split routine: *chest, front* and *side-delts, abs*:

30-degree incline barbell press
100 pounds for 12 slow reps, 120 for 10, 140 for 8
60-degree incline dumbbell press
45 pounds for 12 reps, 50 and 55 for 10
two-arm dumbbell side raises
20 pounds for 12 reps, 25 for 10
one-arm side cable raise
three nonstop sets of 10 reps with 30 pounds

LOWER OUTER/INNER PECS
decline dumbbell press
55 pounds for 12 reps, 60 pounds for 10
dumbbell pullover across bench
60 pounds for 10 reps, 65 pounds for 12

ABS
pulley knee in
35 pounds for 40, 30, then 30 reps
incline leg raise
40, 30, and 30 reps
crunches
50 reps
seated twist
100 reps

BASIC DIET TIPS

It's important to find a lifelong healthy way of eating
without feeling deprived. Before you can correct poor eating habits
you must first become aware of them.
This way you catch the undesirable tendency
before you become comfortable with it.
Simply write down everything you eat today in this diary,
what you ate, how much you ate, and how long it took you to eat it.
Remember: if you eat it, you must write it down.
Observe how you feel before, during, and after eating.
Are you hungry before you eat?
You will get leaner if you experience the onset of hunger before food.
Watch how, what, and how much you eat influences your mood.
Are you happy with the food choices you made today?
How can you improve?

WORKOUT 60

In July of 1985, I spent 40 minutes on an early morning eight-mile bike ride. My arms were all that's left today for this fifth day of my four-way split routine that includes *biceps-triceps-forearms-abs* training. My carb intake that day was only 150 grams ammunition since I was beginning to watch for more definition.

{
face down incline dumbbell curl
  25 pounds for 15 reps, 30 pounds for 12, 35 pounds for 10
dumbbell kickback
  20 pounds for 15 reps, 25 pounds for 12, 30 pounds for 10

{
one-arm dumbbell concentration curl
one-arm dumbbell extension
  three sets of 10 reps with 30, 35, 40 pounds on both exercises

{
preacher cable curl
  90 and 100 pounds for 12 reps
triceps pressdown
  70 and 80 pounds for 10 reps each set

  FOREARMS
{
barbell reverse curl
wrist curl
  both 70 and 80 pounds for 15 reps
grippers
  12 reps

pulley knee in
  three sets of 25 reps with 40 pounds
{
incline leg raise
crunches
one-arm cable crunch
  two sets of 30 reps each

W O R K O U T   6 1

The sixth day of my four-way split routine—*ab-aerobics*—began at sunrise with a 10-mile bike ride in 44 minutes, followed immediately by 480 reps of abs:

GIANT SETTING

{
incline raise
two sets of 40 reps
crunches
two sets of 40 reps
incline knee in
two sets of 40 reps
incline situp
two sets of 40 reps
hanging knee up
two sets of 40 reps
seated twist
two sets of 40 reps

After an hour in my salt water flotation tank, I felt my stored muscular tension diminish. Within the first 10 minutes, the sensation of where my body ends and the tepid salt water begins vanished—as if my body disappeared. I experienced a strong relaxation response when I left the tank; feeling lighter because the body of negativity that had been building all week had gone away leaving me open to fresh perception. Then I spent an hour in the sun as I lay by my pool. That day I again only consumed 150 grams of carbohydrates and less than 50 grams of fats.

L U C I D   D R E A M

Discover a dream in my 1986 diary
being pursued by two adversaries
fleeing I find place to hide
only to have them catch up with me
feeling their threat, travel to another place
and they catch up again so escape
to third place where beautiful high steeples
frame building in front of high mountains
realize there's no place to escape
these two adversaries the dualities, darkness and light
buildings are old, reminiscent of Wilkes College
halls of higher learning, then realizing this is my dream
fight these two adversaries and defeat them
now knowing there's no one to fear nothing to be afraid of
then wake up to chimes blowing in the wind
and roll down umbrellas so they don't blow over at 3:30 A.M..
then go back to bed and dream wise old talking head tells me
OK to train on four way split today like this with two sets or three
of each exercise and slow rhythmic negatives.

FIRST YEAR OF RETIREMENT

Spent the first year of retirement, 1984
healing rotator cuff surgery on December 14, 1983
by Dr. Carter the surgeon
who also fixed Arnold's knee 10 years previously.
This doctor told me he repaired a shoulder hole the size of a half dollar
incurred from a bicycling fall the previous May.
Operation left me with a little scar and a lot of pain
and an arm that shrunk to 13 inches overnight.
Thought I might never train again
but a month later began working out light
and five months hence in good enough shape
to give a posing exhibition 1984 in May.
Anyway, continuing to train, by end of November
with lots of strength regained
training with a partner on a two-way split done every other day
where Day One was calves, thighs, back, and abs
and Day Two chest: shoulders, biceps, triceps, forearms, and abs
on days in between I rode my bike for the same length of time I trained
except when it rained
and on December first rode 22 miles in one hour and 39 minutes.

W O R K O U T   6 2

The next day I began at 7 A.M. with Day One of the two-way split: *calves-thighs-back-abs*. Accompanied by training partner Lynn in my Palm Springs gym, we spent an hour and a half on this routine:

CALVES
standing calf raises
  15 reps with 140 and 160 pounds
donkeys
  200 pounds for 18 reps, 220 for 15
seated calf raises
  two sets of 15 reps with 95 pounds

THIGHS
leg curl
  80 pounds for 12 reps, 90 for 10, 100 for 10
leg extension
  170 pounds for 12 reps, 180 for 11, 190 for 10
Leg Blaster squat
  125 pounds for 12 reps, 145 for 10, 165 for eight

BACK
low cable row
  160, 170, and 180 pounds for 10 reps
T-bar row
  120 and 145 pounds for 10 reps
front pulldown
  10 reps with 170, 180, and 190 pounds
close grip pulldown
  150 and 160 pounds for 10 reps

ABS
{ **pulley knee in**
  incline leg raise
  crunches
    three sets of 30 reps on each
hyperextension
  two sets of 20 reps
seated twist
  100 reps

I LOVED TO RIDE MY BICYCLE

December 3, 1984, rode my bicycle 22
  miles
in one hour 34 and after that
my lower back felt a little sore
so after a few minutes of one leg up
  stretching
I sat by my fireplace, lit a duraflame

warmed up a bit,
enjoyed a real endorphin rush
and felt no pain
reminiscing the 22 miles of road just con-
  quered
so nice to be outdoors and train
aerobically every other day.

MAY 20

W O R K O U T   6 3

At 7 A.M. sharp I met my partner in the gym for Day Two of the hour and a half split routine: *chest-delt-shoulders-biceps-triceps-forearms-abs* workout:

15-degree incline bench barbell press
140 pounds for 10 reps, 160 for nine, 170 for eight
45-degree incline dumbbell press
60 pounds for 10 reps, 65 for eight, 70 for six
75-degree incline dumbbell press
50 pounds for 10 reps, 55 for nine, 60 for seven
decline dumbbell fly
40 pounds for 12 reps, 45 for 11, 50 for 10
dumbbell pullover
60 pounds for 12 reps, 65 for 11, for 70 for 10

BICEPS AND TRICEPS
{
15-degree incline dumbbell curl
30 pounds for 12 reps, 35 for 12, 40 for 10
triceps pressdown
70 pounds for 12 reps, 75 for 11, 80 for 10
{
one-arm dumbbell concentration curl
40 pounds two sets for 10 reps
one-arm dumbbell triceps extension
35 pounds two sets for 10 reps

REAR DELTS
rear cable raise
three sets of 10 reps with 20 pounds
two-arm dumbbell side raises
three sets of 12 reps with 20 pounds

FOREARMS
barbell reverse curl
two sets of 12 reps with 85 pounds

abs exercise
365 total reps on same abs exercises as last workout

At 6:30 the next morning, I rode over 20 miles on my bike for an hour and a half.

DREAM

Dream about women's bodybuilding:
A naked muscular Amazon appeared and
while looking at her, not really sure
should I be envious or
muscle master mind
baiting fishing pole lustful
in a pool of wool or what?
Wake up realizing everything's a metaphor
for something else with no substance in itself.

WORKOUT 64

On December 6, 1984, I worked from 6:00 to 7:40 A.M. with my training partner on *calves-thighs-back-abs*. One of my favorite ways to train calves is to do 15 reps of three different exercises, one right after the other without any rest between (i.e., a tri-set). This gives a tremendous burning sensation in the muscle, which I found to be the secret of calf development—do reps until the onset of a burn.

standing calf raise
120 pounds for 15 reps
seated calf raise
90 pounds for 15 reps
donkey calf raise
200-pound partner sitting on my lower back for 15 reps

rest for three minutes, then do the same tri-set with 10 added pounds on each exercise, holding each rep for five seconds at the top

THIGHS
leg curl
80, 90, and 100 pounds of 10 reps each
leg extension
10 reps with 180, 190, and 200 pounds
Leg Blaster squat
10 reps with 130, 150, and 165 pounds

BACK
T-bar row
120 pounds for 10 reps, 145 for 10, 155 for eight
front pulldown
10 reps with 170, 185, and 195 pounds
close grip pulldown
150 pounds for 10 reps, 160 for nine, 170 for eight

Later I finished with 30 minutes of ab-aerobics at a Zane Haven seminar with eight participants.

LONG EASY BIKE RIDE

Early next morning
rode an easy 20 miles
in one hour forty-five minutes.
Sitting by the pool afterward
reflecting on the satisfaction
from riding all that distance.
I was thankful to have accomplished it safely.
Thinking about all the bike rides I had taken
in the last several years in Palm Springs, Santa Monica,
and cycling in Italy in 1983 and 1984
where townspeople actually applauded as we rode
through town, contrasting to the attitude in Palm Springs
where early morning drivers seem
to almost come after cyclists
and trucks and buses miss me by inches.
The thrill in the danger of it all,
the falls and near misses was it too risky?
Eventually I gave up cycling
after sliding out on a patch of water
bruising my entire right leg.
Now my aerobic activity is walking my dog.
It's a lot safer and puts me outdoors in the early morning
when incredible sunrises
cast interesting shadows
on golden brown mountains.

WORKOUT 65

I got up early to eat a breakfast of oatmeal, fruit, and coffee and give it time enough to digest before working *chest-delts-arms* today. There was no way I wouldn't get a great pump after a carb-loaded breakfast like that. We used the time-star method: concentrating on doing more sets in less time—one hour—rather than using heavier weights. This is the way to build great definition.

CHEST
15-degree incline barbell press
working up to 180 pounds on the third set for six slow reps
40-degree incline dumbbell press
60 pounds for 10 reps, 65 for nine, and 70 for seven
decline fly
40 pounds for 10 reps, 45 for 9, and 50 for eight
dumbbell pullover
65, 70, and 75 pounds for 10 reps
seated dumbbell press
three sets of eight reps with 50 pounds
bent over rear delt cable raise
three sets of 12 reps with 30 pounds
one-arm dumbbell side raise
three sets of 10 reps with 20 pounds

BICEPS AND TRICEPS
{ **incline dumbbell curl**
30 pounds for 12 reps, 40 for 10
pressdowns
two sets of 12 reps with 70 pounds
{ **one-arm dumbbell concentration curl**
40 pounds for two sets of 10
one-arm dumbbell extension
30 pounds for 10 reps, and 35 for eight

FOREARMS
{ **barbell reverse curls**
35 and 40 pounds for 10 reps
barbell wrist curl
two sets of 100 pounds for 15 reps (for a minute couldn't get a grip on anything; still breathless, I did the following tri-set)

ABS
{ **pulley knee-in**
(with 35 pounds)
incline leg raise
crunches
three sets for 35 reps each
hyperextensions
20 reps
seated twists
100 reps

CACTUS METAFOR

Trim a cactus
weeks later new
leaves look back at you
should work your abs, practice
in weeks flabless
ab workouts manifest
slabs written in tablets, rocky ones
word for word
proof, records of progress.
Most important of course
is growing symmetrical cactus
that is bilateral symmetry
means the same on both sides
a mirror image seeing itself always the same
this may be a body's greatest claim to fame
but today ask anybody about symmetry
and they think by mistake
it's some sort of indefinable quality
related to overall harmonious development
when what they really mean to say is
proportion, overall body balance
with no one muscle group attracting
more attention when entire body viewed at once.
You might say every body has relative symmetry
but not every body has proportion
which takes a lifetime to develop
proportion an even greater claim to fame
that's always been my contention.
Symmetry and proportion both important
in bodybuilding as well as in
the art of cactus cultivation
where you must trim the right leaves
for a pleasing finished product.

WORKOUT 66

I trained for the 1983 Mr. Olympia contest with a torn shoulder rotator cuff. So, I couldn't lock out my right arm and had to reduce my upper body weights in training. With limited thinking, I was determined to win it again, or die trying. I almost did by unconsciously inventing a bike accident thus having a graceful exit from the competition. But even though I didn't win, I had the most definition. Here's an early morning *chest-shoulders-back-abs* workout from the summer 1983 contest preparation on my 41st birthday at World Gym in Santa Monica.

dumbbell upright row
25 pounds for 15 reps, 30 for 15, 35 for 12
machine press
70 pounds for 14 reps, 80 for 12, 90 for 10

CHEST
10-degree incline press on Smith machine
100 pounds for 20 reps, 120 for 15, 140 for 10 (not locking out)
dumbbell fly
30, 35, 40, and 45 pounds for 10 to 12 reps
pullover with dumbbells
75, 80, and 85 pounds for 10 to 15 reps

BACK
low cable row
10 reps with 170, 180, and 190 pounds
front pulldown
10 reps with 170, 180, and 190 pounds, then without a break,
one-arm dumbbell row
10 reps with 80, 85, and 90 pounds doing a one-arm lat stretch after each set
close grip pulldown
10 reps with 150, 160, and 170 pounds

My delt-chest-back workout at World Gym was completed, but this was not enough, so I rushed a mile south to Golds Gym in Venice to use their Nautilus machines

torso row (for rear delts and traps)
15 reps with 40, 50, and 60 pounds
behind neck machine (for upper lats)
15 reps with 40, 50, and 60 pounds
two-way chest machine fly
10 reps at 60, 70, and 80 pounds for each two-part movement
chest press
10 reps at 60, 70, and 80 pounds for each two-part movement

ABS
incline leg raise
four sets of 30 reps
Roman chair
four sets of 30 reps
seated twists
100 reps
hyper extensions
20 reps

After finishing at 11:30 A.M., I went home and ate birthday cake.

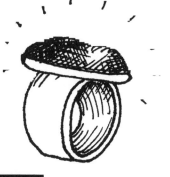

MAY 27

NEW RING

Making up lost time in the sunshine
hematite black bright copper show-stopper
love my whopper ring for a king
made just for me by Christine.

MAY 28

WORKOUT 67

I did this *biceps-triceps-forearms-thighs-calves-abs* workout at World gym on June 29, 1983:

{ **preacher cable curl**
  80 pounds for 12 reps, 90 for 11, 100 for 10
pressdown
  70, 75, and 80 pounds for 10 to 12 reps

{ **one-arm dumbbell concentration curl**
  35, 40, and 45 pounds for 10 to 12 reps

{ **one-arm dumbbell extension**
  30, 35, and 40 pounds for eight to 12 reps

{ **barbell reverse curl**
  65 and 75 pounds for 10 reps
wrist curl
  two sets of 18 reps with an 85-pound barbell

THIGHS

one-legged top extension
  40 pounds for 15 reps, 50 for 12, 60 for 10 to warm up my knees
lunges
  50, 60, and 70-pound barbell for 10 reps
leg curl
  80, 90, and 100 pounds between nine to 12 reps
Leg Blaster squats
  120, 140, and 160 pounds for 10 reps
one-leg curl
  two sets of 15 reps with 30 pounds

CALVES

seated calf raise
  90, 100, and 110 pounds for 15 reps
calf raises on leg press machine
  200, 220, and 240 pounds for 15 reps

ABS

{ **Roman chair situp**
hanging knee ups
  both for three sets of 30 reps
seated twists
  100 reps

EVERYDAY SOUNDS

Back in present time
learning to relax from listening
to everyday sounds like
chirping birds, bouncing ball, sprinkler system
airplane overhead and hearing traffic in the distance
cat meowing, chain saw buzzing
faraway car starting, truck beeping picking up garbage
my dog Tyler playing with his toy, birds chirping all over
some sounds soothing, some annoying
realizing what you hear
can make or ruin your day
choose what you spend your time listening to.
Observe your feeling
when annoying sounds come up
and transform them
by giving them positive meaning.

WORKOUT 68

On July 1, 1983 I rode my bike for 55 minutes before a *delts-chest-back-abs* workout in my Palm Springs gym from 7 to 9 A.M.:

dumbbell upright row
  25 pounds for 20 reps, 30 for 18, 35 for 15
press behind neck
  70 pounds for 15 reps, 85 for 12, 100 for 10
dumbbell rear delt raises
  three sets of 12 reps with 25 pounders
rear cable raise
  20 pounds for three sets of 12 reps
dumbbell fly
  30 pounds for 15 reps, 35 for 12, 40 for 10
pullover
  65 pounds for 15 reps, 70 for 12, 75 for 10

  BACK
low cable row
  160, 170, and 180 pounds for 10 reps
one-arm dumbbell row
  70, 80, and 90 pounds for 10 reps
one-arm lat stretch
front pulldown
  175, 185, and 195 pounds for 10 reps
deadlift
  175 pounds for 10 reps, 215 for nine, 235 for eight

  ABS
pulley knee
  40 pounds for 50, 30, and 20 reps
crunches
  150 reps

THE PRESENT

Change the present
change the future
are you sure you can do it?
Change the present
change the past
but how can you do this
when the present doesn't exist?
Present is a microsecond fiction.

Think you're living in it?
Where is this NOW
when now you see it
now you don't?
Present won't stay
there's just no hope
as time keeps slipping away
it's no joke.

WORKOUT 69

On July 2, 1983, following a 55-minute bike ride after sunrise in the short steep foothills bordering Palm Springs, I did a *calves-thighs-abs* workout for an hour and a half.

CALVES

one legged calf raise (on the Leg Blaster in an upright position)
   first left leg, then right leg, then both legs, 15 reps with 100, 110, and 120 pounds

seated calf raise
   90 pounds for 20 reps, 100 for 16, 115 for 15

leg curl
   80 pounds for 12 reps, 85 for 12, 90 for 10

leg extension
   160 pounds for 12 reps, 180 for 10, 190 for 10

one-leg extension
   60 pounds for 10 reps on each leg

front squat
   80 pounds for 12 reps, 100 for 11, 120 for 10

ABS

incline leg raise
   40, 30, and 30 reps

crunches
   40, 30, and 30 reps

seated twists
   100 reps

one-arm cable crunch with each arm
   two sets of 25 reps

hyperextension
   25 reps

WORKOUT 70

On July 3, 1983 after a 45-minute bike ride, I began *arms-abs* training at 7:10 A.M. in my Palm Springs gym.

{
preacher cable curl
75 pounds for 15 reps, 100 for 14, and 110 for 12
dumbbell kickback face down on the incline bench
15 reps with 25, 30, and 35 pounds

{
one-arm dumbbell concentration curl
10 reps with 35, 40, and 45 pounds
one-arm dumbbell extension
30 pounds for 12 reps, 35 for 11, 40 for 10

{
EZ bar reverse grip preacher curl
35 pounds for 15 reps, 40 for 12, 45 for 10
pressdown
three sets at 75 pounds for 10 reps holding each lock-out one second

FOREARMS
barbell wrist curl
80 pounds for 20 reps, 90 for 15, 100 for 10
wrist rotation
(rotating a two-foot 10-pound bar in each hand for 12, 11, then 10 times)

ABS
pulley knee lying on the floor
45 pounds for 40, 30, 20, and 10 reps resting 20 seconds between sets

{
incline leg raise
three sets of 25
crunches
35, 40, and 50 reps
seated twists (with a pole)
100 reps
one-arm cable crunches
two sets of 20 reps with each arm with 70 pounds

The next day being the Fourth of July, Christine and I drove to Santa Monica and watched the fireworks from the rooftop of our house.

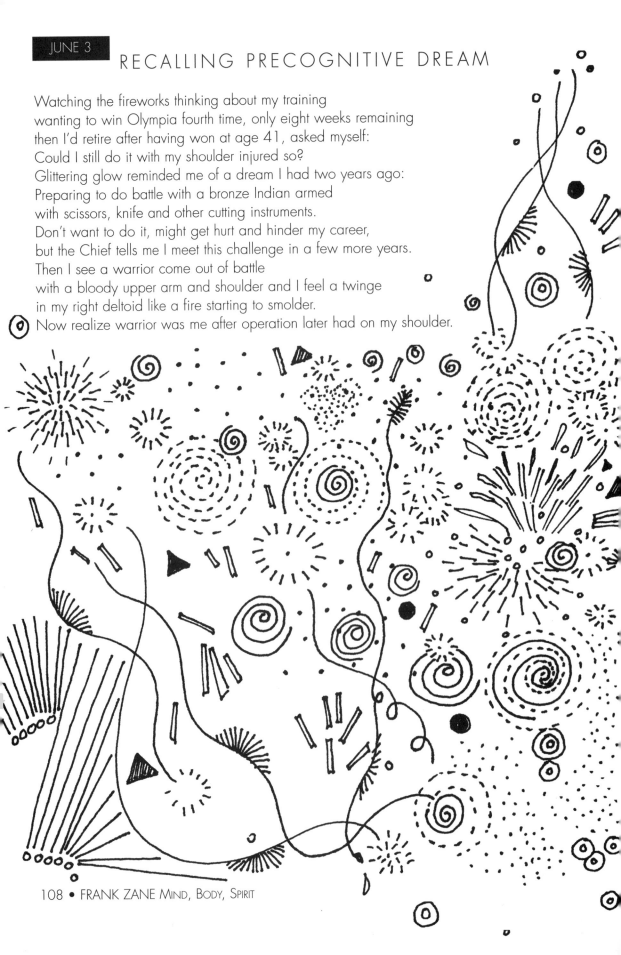

RECALLING PRECOGNITIVE DREAM

Watching the fireworks thinking about my training
wanting to win Olympia fourth time, only eight weeks remaining
then I'd retire after having won at age 41, asked myself:
Could I still do it with my shoulder injured so?
Glittering glow reminded me of a dream I had two years ago:
Preparing to do battle with a bronze Indian armed
with scissors, knife and other cutting instruments.
Don't want to do it, might get hurt and hinder my career,
but the Chief tells me I meet this challenge in a few more years.
Then I see a warrior come out of battle
with a bloody upper arm and shoulder and I feel a twinge
in my right deltoid like a fire starting to smolder.
Now realize warrior was me after operation later had on my shoulder.

WORKOUT 71

Training by myself and thinking about the dream, I figured that at least I can count on me. While doing the low incline press on the Smith machine, I remembered how I couldn't lockout because my shoulder hurt. I thought it was just a sprain but later found out it was almost a complete tear in the rotator cuff. Well, that explained all the pain. But I knew I had to train, so I got into a *delts-chest-back* training in the World Gym at 9 A.M..

dumbbell upright row
25 pounds for 15 reps, 35 for 12, 40 for 10
machine press
70 pounds for 15 reps, 80 for 12, 90 for 10

CHEST
incline barbell press
100 pounds for 15 reps, 120 for 10, 140 for eight with slow negatives
dumbbell flys
35, 40, and 45 pounds for 12 reps each
dumbbell pullover
80 pounds for 15 reps, 85 for 12 reps, 90 for 10

BACK
front pulldown
180 pounds for 12 reps, 190 for 11, 200 for 10
low cable row
180 pounds for 10 reps, 190 for 10, 200 for 10
one-arm dumbbell row
80, 90, and 100 pounds for 10 reps (followed by a one-arm lat stretch)
close grip pulldown
160, 170, and 180 pounds for 10 reps

DELTS
behind neck machine
40, 50, and 60 pounds for 15 reps for lats (using the Nautilus™ machines at Golds Gym)
torso row
50, 60, and 70 pounds for 15 reps each set
Nautilus two-way chest machine
80 pounds for 12 reps, 90 for 10, and 100 for eight

ABS
Roman chair situp
75, 50, and 50 reps
hanging knee ups
three sets of 25 reps
incline leg raises
three sets of 20 reps
flat out on seated twist
100 reps
hyperextensions
two sets of 20 reps
bike riding
up San Vicente Boulevard for 34 minutes with Christine

ANOTHER DREAM

That night had another dream
in it I see Lee Haney
doing one-arm dumbbell row with one leg kneeling
on a bench and he has wires
connected to all the muscles on the left side
of his body almost as if he's a puppet on strings
and as he fires off rep after rep with a 150-pound dumbbell I see
his lats swell like a pair of wings
looking back didn't know he'd place ahead of me
number three Mr. Olympia in Munich, Germany.

WORKOUT 72

From 8:20 to 10:40 A.M. on July 6, I did *arms-legs-abs* training at the World Gym:

ARMS
{
preacher cable curl
70 pounds for 12 reps, 80 for 12, 90 for 10
dumbbell kickback
30 pounds for three sets of 10 reps
}

{
one-arm dumbbell concentration curl
35, 40, and 45 pounds for 10 reps
one-arm dumbbell extension
35 pounds for 10 reps, 40 for eight, 40 for nine
pressdown
three sets of 10 reps with 80 pounds
alternate dumbbell curl
10 reps with 35, 40, and 45 pounds
}

{
EZ bar reverse grip preacher curl
three sets with 55 pounds for eight reps
barbell wrist curl
three sets 85 pounds for 15 to 20 reps
}

THIGHS
one leg top extension
40 pounds for 15 reps, 50 for 12, 60 for nine
lunges with Leg Blaster
50 pounds for 12 reps, 60 for 11, 70 for 10
leg curl
80 pounds for 12 reps, 90 for 10, 100 for 8
hack squats (using a light weight for a pump)
40 pounds for 12 reps, 60 for 11, 80 for 10

CALVES
standing calf raises
200, 220, and 240 pounds for 15 reps
seated calf raises
100, 110, and 120 pounds for 15 reps
calf raises on the leg press machine
four sets of 15 reps at 250 pounds

ABS
{
hanging knee ups
four sets of 30 reps
Roman chair situp
30, 30, 30, and 50 reps
}
seated twists
100 reps
hyperextension
two sets of 20 reps

SUNBATHING

Arrived early in Palm Springs and after eating a spinach mushroom omelet
for breakfast went out by my pool and got a few hours of sun
floating on a raft in the water made me feel cool
enough to withstand the heat
as the temperature climbed to 110 degrees by noon
when it got too hot went inside and felt much cooler
then wrote all afternoon on my computer.

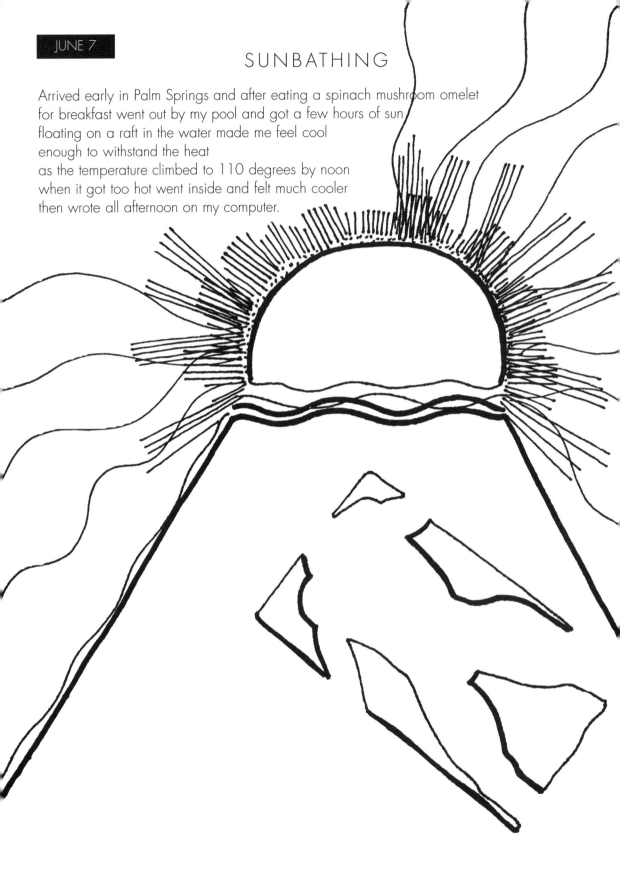

WORKOUT 73

The next day after riding my bike for 48 minutes, I trained *delts-chest-back* from 6:50 to 9 A.M. in my Palm Springs gym.

DELTS

dumbbell upright row
25 pounds for 20 reps, 30 for 15, 35 for 12, 40 for 12

press behind neck with barbell
80 pounds for 14 reps, 95 for 12, 105 for 10

dumbbell raise to the rear
three sets of 25 pounds for 12 reps

rear delt cable raise
10 pounds for 15, 15 pounds for eight, 15 pounds for eight

one-arm side cable raise
two sets of 12 with 20 pounds nonstop with each arm

CHEST

dumbbell fly
35 pounds for 12 reps, 40 for 12, 45 for 10

tensing pecs
15 seconds between sets to bring out inner pec striations

pullover
70, 75, and 80 pounds for 10 reps each

BACK

front pulldown
180, 190, and 200 pounds all for 10 reps

low cable row
180, 190, and 200 pounds for 10 reps was as heavy as I could go

one-arm dumbbell row
90, 95, and 100 all for 10 reps

deadlift
195 pounds for 10, 235 pounds for nine, 255 pounds for seven (I used straps with a wide grip)

ABS

pulley knee-in
40 pounds for 50, 30, and 20 reps

{ **incline leg raise**
crunches
four sets of 25 reps

seated twist
100 reps

hyperextension
25 and 15 reps

WORKOUT 74

After riding my bike for 50 minutes during the pre-dawn hours before it got hot, I began an *abs-calves-thighs* workout at 7:10 A.M.:

ABS
incline leg raise
100 reps
crunches
100 reps
seated twist
100 reps

CALVES
one leg calf raise with Leg Blaster
90, 100, and 110 pounds for 15 reps
seated calf raise
18 reps at 100, 105, and 110 pounds
standing Leg Blaster calf raises
200 pounds for 15 reps

THIGHS
leg curl
80 pounds for 12 reps, 90 for 10, 100 for 10
leg extension
160 pounds for 10 reps, 180 for 10, 200 for nine
one-leg top extension
60 pounds for 15 reps with each leg
sissy squats on Leg Blaster
three sets of 15 reps with 100 pounds

WORKOUT 75

At 7 A.M. I was in my gym on July 10, 1983, to work on *arms-abs* after riding my bike for 40 minutes.

ARMS
{ **preacher cable curl**
  80 pounds for 12 reps, 90 for 10, 80 for 10
dumbbell kickback
  25 pounds for 20 reps, 30 for 15, 35 for 12
{ **one-arm dumbbell concentration curl**
one-arm dumbbell extension
  35 pounds for 10 reps, 40 for nine, 45 for eight both
  exercises
{ **alternate dumbbell curl**
  40 pounds for 10 reps, 45 for nine, 50 for eight
pressdown
  75 pounds for 12 reps, 80 for 11, 85 for 10

then took a quick drink of water

FOREARMS
{ **reverse barbell curl**
  10 reps at 80 and 90 pounds
barbell wrist curl
  80 pounds for 18 reps, 90 for 15
squeezing two grippers
  two sets of 20 reps each (afterwards, I shook out my
  hands for 10 seconds)

ABS
pulley knee in
  45 pounds strapped around my ankles for 50, 30, and
  20 reps
{ **incline leg raise**
  40, 30, and 30 reps
crunches
  three sets of 40 reps
seated twist
  three sets of 50 reps
hyperextension
  25 then 15 reps

After that, I had breakfast and laid in the sun.

CYCLING AND SUNBATHING

The next day I rested, well almost anyway
urgency told me to get more definition
so I rode bike 35 minutes and then sunbathed for two hours.
By this time I was getting quite a tan.
Man, it got so hot in Palm Springs in July
not a soul to be seen in town around noon
and I can understand why since it was 118 degrees
but I knew a dark tan was essential for competition
and I gradually got darker and darker
applying Vaseline on my nose and lips to prevent burning
and moisturizer after I came out of the sun
and made sure to never get a sunburn.

WORKOUT 76

Arriving yesterday afternoon in Santa Monica and went shopping in the mall where all eyes were on this large muscled man sporting a well-worn Gold's Gym tank top torn, multi-colored shoes, and clown pants. Next morning at 7A.M.I saw him at Gold's Gym in Venice hogging the dumbbells while leaving the heaviest ones lying all over the floor. Luckily, he left the lighter ones alone which I used to train *delts and chest*.

DELTS
dumbbell upright row
25, 30, and 35 pounds for 20 reps
rear delt machine
60 pounds for 12 reps, 70 for 10, 80 for 10
machine front press
60 pounds for 15 reps, 85 for 12, 100 for 10, 115 for seven

CHEST
incline barbell press
100 pounds for 12 reps, 120 for 10, 140 for eight
pec deck
100 pounds for 10 reps, 110 for 10, 120 for eight

Then I drove to World gym and worked on *back and abs* from 8:15 to 9:30 A.M..

front pulldown
190 pounds for 10 reps, 200 for 10, 210 pounds for eight reps
cable crossover behind neck
40, 50, and 60 pounds for 15 reps
two-arm lat stretch
low cable row
180 pounds for 10 reps, 190 for 10, 200 for eight
one-arm dumbbell row
90, 95, and 100 pounds for 10 reps each
one-arm lat stretch
close grip pulldown
150 pounds for 10 reps, 160 for 10, 170 for eight

ABS
Roman chair situp
100 reps
hanging knee up
40, 30, and 30 reps
{ **incline leg raise**
crunches
four sets of 25 each
seated twists
100 reps
hyperextension
25 reps
walking
fast for a quarter mile

DISCIPLINED SUFFERING

Sometimes several hours
after a shoulder workout
my deltoids were so sore
couldn't raise my arms
more than a few inches
but since soreness
intense only in deltoids
I could tolerate it

deltoids wouldn't be exercised
again for at least 24 hours
in which time they'd rest, recuperate,
 repair
as I prepared for the next training session
thinking about how I
make my body suffer
in a controlled way.

JUNE 14

W O R K O U T   7 7

I awoke 6:30 A.M., and had branched chain amino acids with six ounces carrot juice followed by a breakfast of spinach mushroom omelet, four ounces cottage cheese, and eight ounces of coffee sweetened with glycine. At 8:40 A.M. I began a *leg* workout at World Gym.

calf raise on leg press machine
 250 pounds for 20 reps, 260 for 18, 270 for 16
seated calf raise
 16 reps with 100, 110, and 120 pounds
standing calf raises
 16 reps with 220, 240, and 260 pounds

 THIGHS
leg curl
 80 pounds for 12 reps, 90 for 10, 100 for 10
lunges
 60, 70, and 80 pounds of 10 reps
leg extension
 160 pounds for 12 reps, 180 for 10, 200 for eight
hack squat
 40 pounds for 15 reps, 50 for 12, 60 for 10

 ABS
Roman chair situp
 200 reps
hanging knee up
 four sets of 25 reps
seated twist
 100 reps
hyperextension
 25 then 15 reps

After which I went home, ate lunch, went to the beach, laid in the sun, body surfed in the waves, and had fun.

NO STRESS?

If you think you've got no stress
then you may have guessed wrong
because that could be just stressed repressed,
unconsciously buried deep down inside
stress can manifest itself
as headaches at best or accidents.
As Carl Jung once said,
"When an inner situation is not made
conscious the result appears as fate."

JUNE 16

WORKOUT 78

After breakfast on July 14, 1983, I started *arm* training at 8:30 A.M. at World Gym.

{ **alternate dumbbell curl**
    40, 45, and 50 pounds for 10 reps
dumbbell kickback
    30, 35, and 40 pounds for 10 reps

{ **one-arm dumbbell concentration curl**
    40, 45, and 50 pounds for 10 reps
one-arm dumbbell extension
    35, 40, and 45 pounds for 10 reps

{ **preacher cable curl**
    80, 90, and 100 pounds for 10
pressdown
    70, 80, and 90 pounds for 10 reps

FOREARMS
{ **barbell reverse wrist curl**
    30, 35, and 40 pounds for 10 reps
barbell wrist curl
    three sets using 100 pounds for 15 reps

Because my forearms were so pumped, I had to shake my hands for half a minute.

ABS
Roman chair situp
    150 reps
incline leg raise
    40, 30, and 30 reps with 20 seconds rest between sets
seated twists
    100 reps
hyperextension
    25 and 15 reps

After the workout ate crab and trout with Christine at our favorite restaurant on Pacific Palisades beach.

WORKOUT 79

With a posing exhibition only a few days away, I felt the need to work on *abs* and *legs* without squatting with heavy weights which blurs thigh definition when done too close to an exhibition. So I did three tri-sets on each body part in a workout lasting about one hour. This is tough, but it builds great definition and endurance.

ABS
{
hanging knee ups
three sets of 30 reps
crunches
three sets of 30 reps
seated twist
three sets of 40 reps
}

THIGHS
{
leg extension
170, 180, and 190 pounds for 12 reps
leg curl
80, 90, and 100 pounds for 12 reps
stairclimber
three sets of two minutes apiece
}

CALVES
{
standing calf raise with Leg Blaster
140 and 160 pounds for 15 reps
seated calf raise
15 reps of 90 and 100 pounds
donkeys
three sets of 20 reps with 215-pound rider
}

DAY BEFORE TRAVEL

Packed for tomorrow's trip
then got two hours of sun
and visualized my posing routine
saw myself doing each pose
while listening to my posing music
on an audio cassette with headphones.
Later in the day, practiced my posing routine
to the music for half an hour.
Ate 200 grams of carbohydrate today
200 grams of protein (had a lean filet mignon
which helped my strength)
60 grams of fat, mostly from lecithin and
a little olive oil for a daily total of a little over 2100 calories.

POSING EXHIBITION

The next day Friday July 15th
caught a plane for Santa Rosa, California
to give a posing exhibition in pretty good shape
and while there had this dream:
The path ran parallel to a stream
meandering through woods and led
to a large open field.
As I watched, a giant placed a golden ball
on a large tee hitting it several thousand meters
with the golf club he wielded
then he invited me
to follow him into the field
the giant retrieved the ball
and handed it to me.
Placing the ball on one of my small tees
I hit it into a pond 100 meters away with my club.
As the ball sank to the bottom of the pond
the hairy giant said
"To retrieve your golden ball
you must dive to the bottom of the pond
then place the ball on this long tall tee instead.
It's impossible to drive the ball
out of the pond with the small tees
you've been using.
That's why you're losing."
Then the giant pulled some hair
from his chest and handed it to me
then he hit the ball a mile high in the air.
Awakening, I asked
"What is the meaning of the tees and the hairy giant's hair?"

AT THE PHYSIQUE CONTEST

Saturday the next day
waking up, as I lay
in bed, visualizing my posing routine
saw myself getting in better and better condition
then called a friend and
he and his girlfriend came up to see me.
Felt elated posing to the audience ovation.

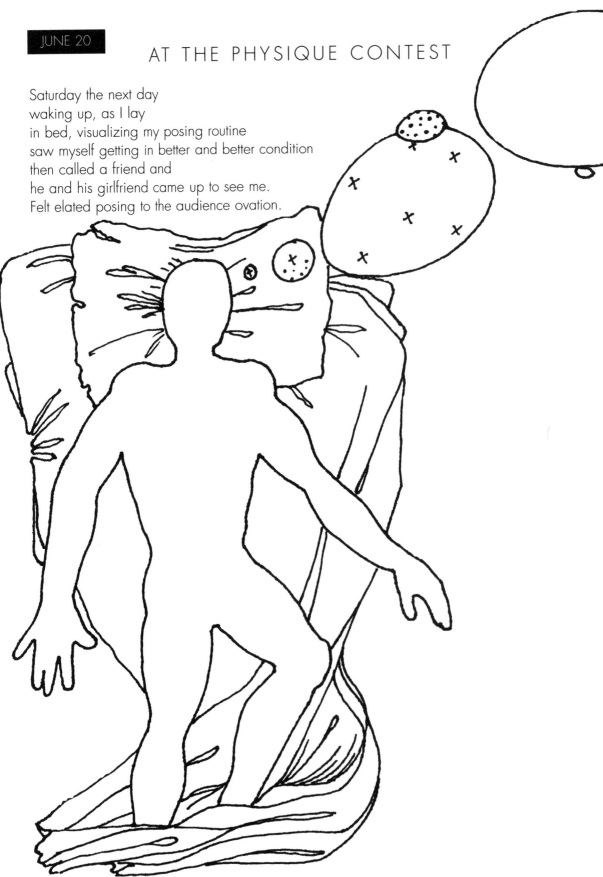

SPRING TRAINING IN RETROSPECT

Looking back on this spring's training—some recent and some from the past—it's vital to recognize importance of continuity with a regular pattern.

DATE	MY WORKOUT	YOUR WORKOUT
Mar 21	upper body, abs	
Mar 23	thighs, calves, aerobics	
Mar 25	stretching, abs	
Mar 27	chest, shoulders, triceps, abs, aerobics	
Mar 30	biceps, triceps, forearms	
April 1	thighs, calves, aerobics, abs	
April 4	chest, shoulders, triceps, aerobics, abs	
April 6 -	back, biceps, forearms, abs	
April 8	thighs, calves, abs, aerobics	
April 10	chest, shoulders, triceps, abs, aerobics	
April 12	back, biceps, forearms, abs, aerobics	
April 14	aerobics	
April 16	chest, shoulders, triceps	
April 19	back, biceps, forearms, abs	
April 22	thighs, calves, abs	
April 24	chest, shoulders, triceps, abs	
April 27	back, biceps, forearms, aerobics	
April 29	thighs, calves, abs	
May 1	chest, shoulders, triceps, aerobics, abs	
May 3	abs, back, biceps, forearms, aerobics	
May 5	thighs, calves, ab-aerobics	
May 7	aerobics, abs, chest, shoulders, triceps	
May 9	aerobics, back, shoulders, abs	
May 10	abs, calves, thighs	
May 12	chest, shoulders, abs	
May 14	aerobics, biceps, triceps, forearms, abs	

May 15	aerobics, abs
May 17	aerobics
May 18	calves, thighs, back, abs
May 19	aerobics
May 20	chest, shoulders, biceps, triceps, fore arms, abs
May 22	calves, thighs, back, ab-aerobics
May 23	aerobics
May 24	chest, shoulders, biceps, triceps, fore arms, abs
May 26	chest, shoulders, back, abs
May 28	biceps, triceps, forearms, thighs, calves, abs
May 30	aerobics, shoulders, chest, back, abs
June 1	aerobics, calves, thighs, abs
June 2	aerobics, biceps, triceps, abs
June 4	shoulders, chest, back, ab-aerobics
June 6	biceps, triceps, forearms, thighs, calves, abs
June 8	aerobics, shoulders, chest, back, abs
June 9	aerobics, abs, calves, thighs
June 10	biceps, triceps, forearms, abs
June 11	aerobics
June 12	chest, shoulders, back abs
June 14	calves, thighs, abs
June 16	biceps, triceps, forearms, abs
June 17	abs, thighs, calves
June 18	practice posing
June 20	posing exhibition

And still thinking of spring
I remember what Thoreau wrote
as Walden passages ring familiar:

Why should we be in such desperate haste to succeed,
and in such desperate enterprises?
If a man does not keep pace with his companions,
perhaps it is because he hears a different drummer.
Let him step to the music he hears,
however measured or far away.
It is not important that he should mature as soon
as an apple tree or an oak.
Shall he turn his spring into summer?
If the condition of things which we were made for is not yet,
what were any reality which we can substitute?

Every man is the builder of a temple, called his body,
to the god he worships, after a style purely his own,
nor can he get off by hammering marble instead.
We are all sculptors and painters,
and our material is our own flesh and blood and bones.
Any nobleness begins at once to refine a man's features,
any meanness...to imbrute them.

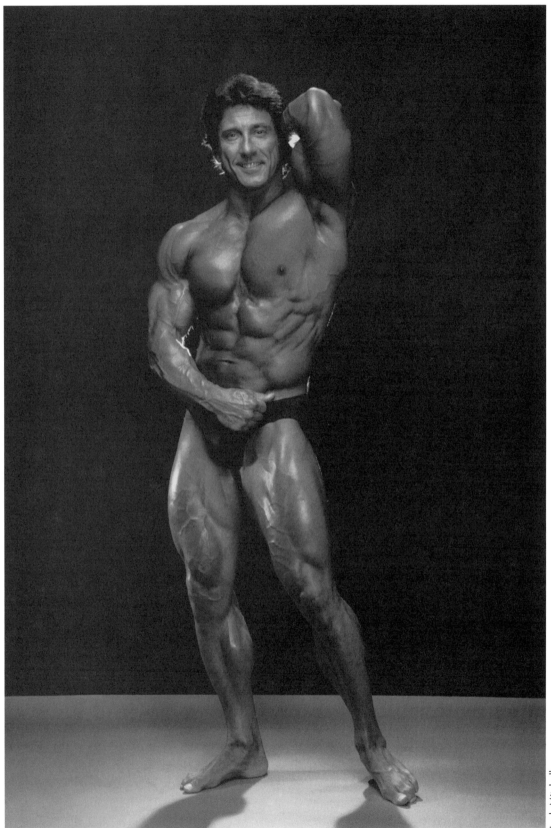

SUMMER DIARY

Noumena
or what I see
eyes closed is a painting
two dimensionally
a sculpture
dimensions of three
a moving being
streaking through
the fourth dimension of time
extension into space
all over the place
with room in me for a timeless life
full of hunger, thirst, work
my dog and my wife.

BODY ART HIGHEST

The highest art form is the human body
expressing who we are and ought to be.
This my personal ongoing creation
through scientific training gaining mastery
a quest for personal meaning, eventually
this matter/spirit dichotomy complex interwoven fabric
becomes clear momentarily looking through past diaries
what I'd like to do is to continue
giving a progressive program increasing
in intensity, making training more demanding.
When I was younger, did a lot more than I need to do now,
It was a lot of overtraining but after all, I was competing.
Now I remember parsimony rules:
get the most from the least, don't be fooled
more is not better necessarily.

WORKOUT 80

Riding a bike over 20 miles every other day burns a lot of calories. But in 1977—declared by my ad in Muscle & Fitness magazine as the "Year of Zane"—I did no formal aerobics because I weight-trained twice a day. For example, on August 16 of that year, my friend Ulf and I did this *back-biceps-forearms* workout at World Gym:

bent over barbell rowing
140 pounds for 12 reps, 160 for 12, and 180 for 10
one-arm dumbbell row
three sets of 10 reps with 95 pounds
pulldown behind neck
190 pounds for three sets of 10 reps
front chin
three sets of 10 reps
barbell curl
90 pounds for 12 reps, 110 for 10, and 120 for eight
alternate dumbbell curl
50 pounds for 10 reps, 55 for eight, 60 for six
low incline dumbbell curl
three sets of 10 reps with 35 pounds
preacher curls
70 pounds for three sets of 10 reps
reverse barbell curl
90, 100, and 100 pounds for 10 reps
barbell wrist curl
90, 100, and 100 pounds for 15 reps

ABS
hanging knee-ups
four sets of 25 reps

LARRY SCOTT FAN

Thinking back to when I was a big fan
of Larry Scott in the 60s and 70s
and this imperial bodybuilding idol
1965-66 affixed Olympia crown two times.
The world and beyond transfixed
delts and arms like his have never been since.
Remember staring in the mirror
and see his deltoided appendages
in my imagination instead of mine
as part of my visualization exercise
on me they looked fine.

WORKOUT 81

That same afternoon August 16 in 1977, I did a *thighs-calves-abs* workout.

leg extension
80 pounds for 16 reps, 90 for 14, 100 for 12 (Joe Gold's unusual machine limited our weights)

squats
three sets of 15 reps with 185 pounds

hack machine
three sets of 10 reps with 100 pounds

leg curl
40 pounds for 18 reps, 50 for 14, 60 for 12 (which was about half of what could be used on my Nautilus leg curl)

CALVES

calf raise on leg press machine
four sets of 15 reps with 180 pounds

seated calf raises
three sets of 15 reps with 115, 135, and 145 pounds

ABS

Roman chair situps
100 reps

incline knee
40, 30, and 30 reps

hyperextension
20 reps

RHEO BLAIR

1970s good old days, can't help thinking of Rheo Blair.
Short stature, pompadour of black wavy hair
grand piano playing singing songs baritone
was his form of vocal training.
He was adept at swinging on monkey bars attached to his ceiling and
we'd sit there for hours on bean bag chairs
waiting for our supplements, eating protein ice cream bars.
Rheo died years ago. He knew more about
amino acids and vitamins than anyone else.

WORKOUT 82

For an hour and 20 minutes on August 17, 1977, I worked on *delts-chest-triceps* with my partner Ulf, Mr. Sweden, at World Gym in Santa Monica:

TRAPS
dumbbell upright row
15 reps for 40, 45, and 50 pounds
dumbbell shrug
80 pounds for 15 reps, 90 for 12, and 100 for 10

DELTS
seated dumbbell press
60 pounds for 12 reps, 65 for 10, 70 for eight
dumbbell side raises
25 pounds for 12 reps, 30 for 11, 35 for 10

CHEST
incline dumbbell flys
65 pounds for 12 reps, 70 for 11, 75 for 10 (that became more like presses on our last sets)
decline dumbbell flys
10 reps with 65, 70, and 75 pounds
dumbbell pullover
95 pounds for four sets of 10 reps

TRICEPS
close grip bench press
10 reps with 170, 180, and 190 pounds
one-arm dumbbell extension
10 reps with 35, 40, and 45 pounds
pressdown
10 reps with 75, 80, and 85 pounds

ABS
Roman chair situp
150 reps
incline knee-ups
40, 30, and 30 reps
hyperextensions
20 reps

CHRISTINE SILVER GEMSTONE QUEEN

Sitting upstairs writing
while Christine's down there
in her studio soldering making jewelry
necklaces, rings beautiful things out of
    silver
and gemstones galore
amethyst, blue topaz, turquoise, black onyx
hematite, Mexican fire opals, delight in
rhodochrosite
and in lapis lazuli I see a little of heaven
looking at the birthday ring she made me
at half past seven
an amazing woman
sometimes she's tired working so hard
always inspired thinking of her
I hear Tyler barking in the front yard.

WORKOUT 83

On August 31, 1977, I met with Ulf at World Gym to begin our *back-biceps-forearms-abs* training at 9 A.M.:

BACK

barbell rowing
140 pounds for 12 reps, 160 for 10, 180 for 10, and 190
for 10 (being careful not to let the bar hit our knees)

dumbbell rowing one-arm
95, 100, and 105 pounds for 10 reps

low cable row
150, 160, and 170 pounds for 10 reps

pulldown behind neck
10 reps with 190, 190, and 200 pounds

stiff arm pulldown
70 and 80 pounds for 10 reps

BICEPS

low incline dumbbell curl
35 pounds for 12 reps, 40 for 10, 45 for eight

preacher curl
three sets of 10 reps with 70 pounds

one-arm dumbbell concentration curl
three sets of eight reps with 40-pounder

FOREARMS

{
barbell reverse curl
three sets of 10 reps with 80 pounds

barbell wrist curl
three sets of 20 reps with 100 pounds

ABS

Roman chair situp
100 reps

incline knee-in
40, 30, and 30 reps

MY PHILOSOPHY
OF BODYBUILDING—1977

Degree of development is directly proportional
to concentration while training.
Discipline is necessary to succeed in bodybuilding
and useful in overcoming life's problems
a means to personal growth, personality development
method to resolve Narcissus complex.
It's not like I'm fascinated by what I see in the mirror.
Bodybuilding compensates for lack of attention in formative years
since the feelings and behaviors learned as a child persist into adulthood
even though the reasons for these actions no longer exist.
What bodybuilders really need and want is attention and appreciation.
To me bodybuilding is a science of introspection,
looking into the body deeper and deeper, studying the self.
When younger I wanted to be a scientist.
Mirror is an exercise in looking at yourself.
Look for flaws, imperfections
from image as you are, build your perfect body.
Visualize yourself as you want to be realistically.
Bodybuilding can teach how to look at your shortcomings.
As you begin to notice them in your body
and start seeing them in your personality
watch yourself project them on to others.
Seems most successful bodybuilders come from disciplining parents.
Strict discipline plus not enough attention from my father as I grew
I knew lack of attention from my peers led me to being by myself a lot.
Used to practice shooting basketball, this sport was about centering.
In Boy Scouts four years attaining rank of Eagle Scout.
Got all A's in high school graduated class valedictorian.
Not lifting a log at Philmont Scout Ranch in New Mexico
motivated me to take up bodybuilding.
Discovering bodybuilding and archery at same time age 14,
later found out about yoga and meditation at 16.
Did hatha yoga breath control read Patanjali
and became fascinated by Siddhis, miraculous special powers
attained through concentration and meditation and became more focused.
Third contest ever entered age 18 won third in Teen Age Mr. America
proud of trophy now I had three, went to Chuck Robbins
sporting goods store to get it inscribed and a fat guy age 30 told me
when I got to his age I'd look like him or even worse, told the man
I'd never look like him, nothing more miraculous than
the human body developed to proportioned symmetrical muscular potential
paying attention to details of each exact movement of exercises
enabled me to transform my body in a way that was gradual.

WORKOUT 84

Later on August 31, 1977, at 3:30 P.M. I was alone in the gym for a thighs-calves-abs workout. Afterwards Christine and I would go see a Rudolph Nureyev ballet at the Greek Theater in Los Angeles.

THIGHS

leg extension
70 pounds for 20 reps, 80 for 15, 90 for 10, 100 for 10 (could have done over twice this on a Nautilus)

squats
135 pounds for 15 reps, and 185, 205, and 225 pounds for 10 reps

hack machine
three sets of 10 reps for 105 pounds

one-legged curl
(quit after one set because my ankle was bleeding from an Achilles tendon cut)

CALVES

donkeys
220 pounds five sets of 25 to 30 reps

seated calf raises
100 pounds for four sets of 15 reps (I should have rested longer between sets but I paid no heed to this cowardly advice from calves)

incline face down calf raise on hack machine
195 pounds for three sets of 15 reps

standing raises
240 pounds for two sets of 15 reps

ABS

crunches
40, 30, and 30 reps

hanging knee ups
30, 25, and 25 reps

hyperextension
20 reps

TODAY

Modern day transistor mystic
practice right speech.
Problem today is
talk is cheap
but eventually
you will pay
for what you say.
It's always that way.

WORKOUT 85

It was September 1, just one month before the 1977 Mr. Olympia contest. I trained at World Gym with my friend Ulf on *delts-chest-triceps* workout:

TRAPS

dumbbell upright row
40 pounds for 15 reps, 45 for 10, 50 for 10

dumbbell press
65 pounds for 12 reps, 70 for 11, 75 for 10

one dumbbell front raise
50, 55, and 60, pounds for 10 reps

dumbbell side raise
25, 30, and 35 pounds for 10 reps

REAR DELTS

rear delt face down incline dumbbell raises
30-pounders for three sets of 10 reps

bent over cable raises
15 pounds three sets of 10 reps

machine front presses
120, 130, and 130 pounds for 10 reps (my rear delts hurt so much had to rub them with liniment)

CHEST

bench press
135 pounds for 15 reps, 185 for 12, 225 for 10

incline dumbbell presses
70 pounds for 10 reps, 75 for 10, 80 for nine

decline flies
three sets of 10 reps with 50-pound dumbbells

dumbbell pullover
three sets at 85 pounds for 10 reps

cable crossover
three sets of 10 reps with 35 pounds

TRICEPS

close grip bench press
135 pounds for 10, eight, and seven reps (with only 45 seconds rest between sets)

pressdown
80 pounds for three sets 10 reps

EZ bar overhead extension
three sets of eight reps with 85 pounds

dumbbell kickback
three sets of 10 reps with 30 pounds

ABS

Roman chair
100 reps

incline knee-in
40, 30, and 30 reps

crunches
two sets of 40

hyperextention
20 reps

POWER OF SUSTAINED CONCENTRATION

No mind wandering or conversation during sets or in between
moving rapidly making each set really count
not resting more than one minute in between
barely catching your breath amounts
to cultivating the breathless state
pacing the floor stretching
workout is one giant set of exercises breathing me.
Train like this and get in real shape.

JULY 4

WORKOUT 86

On September 9, 1977, I met my partner at World Gym at nine in the morning to begin what I recorded in my journal as the best *back-biceps-forearms* training, yet.

front pulldown
  10 reps with 170, 180, and 190 pounds
bent over barbell rowing
  10 reps with 130, 150, and 170 pounds
one-arm dumbbell row
  10 reps with 90, 100, and 110 pounds
low cable row
  160 pounds for 10 reps, 170 for nine, 180 for eight
pulldown behind neck
  10 reps with 180, 190, and 200 pounds
stiff arm pulldown
  three sets of 10 reps using 80 pounds

  BICEPS
dumbbell concentration curl
  35 pounds for 10 reps, 40 for eight, 45 for eight
curled dumbbells on low incline
  10 reps with 30, 35, and 40 pounds
preacher cable curl
  90 pounds for three sets of 10 reps
alternate dumbbell curls
  50 pounds for three sets of eight reps

  FOREARMS
barbell reverse curl
  three sets of 10 reps with 70 pounds
wrist curl
  three sets of 15 reps with 100-pound barbell

  ABS
Roman chair situp
  200 reps
seated twist
  100 reps
crunches
  100 nonstop reps

W O R K O U T   8 7

Septeptember 12 in 1977, I trained *thighs and calves* in the following way.

THIGHS
leg extension (on Joe Gold's hard leg extension machine)
60 pounds for 20 reps, 70 for 15, 80 for 12, 90 for 10
one leg extension
40 pounds for 15 reps (I hated this machine because it sometimes hurt my knee)
squat (wrapping my knees between sets)
135, 185, 225, 245, and 265 pounds for 10 reps
leg press
190, 210, and 230 pounds for 12 reps
leg curl
50 pounds for 15 reps, 60 for 12, 70 for 10

CALVES
standing calf machine
15 reps with 200, 240, and 260 pounds
seated calf raise
100, 110, and 120 pounds for 15 reps
donkey calf raises
three sets of 18 to 20 reps (because I paused at the top of each rep, my calves felt numb afterwards)

PRESENCE

Presence means being there
wherever you are
fully in the moment.
It means being there totally
in what you are doing
not stuck in flashbacks of the past
or speculation about the future
but totally in the now
you sure will be powerful
just admit
you can do it.

WORKOUT 88

Feeling very tired on September 13, 1977, I forced myself to train from 9:10 to 10:45 A.M. on *chest–triceps–abs*. Later that afternoon after a good rest, I returned for *delts*. I remember being tired and my calves feeling really sore as I went home that day.

CHEST
incline dumbbell press
60, 70, and 80 pounds for 10 reps
bench press
135, 185, 225, and 235 pounds for 10 reps
decline dumbbell flys
50, 55, 60 pounds for 10 reps
dumbbell pullover
80, 90, and 100 pounds for 10 reps
cable crossover
three sets of 25 pounds for 12 reps

TRICEPS
close grip bench press on the Smith machine
135, 140, and 145 pounds for 10 reps
pressdown
80, 85, and 90 pounds for 10 reps
lying triceps extension
80, 90, and 100 pounds for 10 reps
one-arm dumbbell extension
35, 40, and 45 for eight to 10 reps

ABS
Roman chair situp
200 reps
seated twist
100 reps (for a break, I went home, ate, took a nap, returned to the gym)

CALVES
incline hack machine face down calf raises
five sets of 20 reps

DELTS
dumbbell upright row
45 pounds for four sets 10 reps
dumbbell press
10 reps with 60, 70, and 75 pounds
two dumbbell front raises
10 reps with 30, 35, and 40 pounds
seated side dumbbell raises
three sets of 10 reps with 25 pounds
seated dumbbell rear delt raises
three sets of 12 reps with 25 pounds
rear cable raises
three sets of 10 reps with 20 pounds

ABS
{ **incline knee-in**
crunches
both for 40, 30, and 30 reps
hyperextension
20 reps

SYMBOLIC DREAM OF WINNING

About two weeks before the 1977 Mr. Olympia had a dream
down on Venice beach Robbie Robinson throws a long spiral pass
with a football 80 yards then a kid throws a pass even longer
without trying too hard the football hit the hangar where
Robbie's model airplane is stored, it explodes.
Looking back now I know what this means
and realize this kid was me.
Remember that year Robbie looked incredible
two weeks before the show, round, wide and muscular
everybody said no way I could win it but instead
paying no attention to this kept training, tensing, posing
and knew the contest wasn't between him and me
it was between me and me, it was about how good
I could be so I went all out in my training
and two weeks before the contest
I passed into the "point of no return":
That is one day looking in the mirror
noticed a dramatic improvement in my muscularity.
Everyday after that it got more and more impressive
gaining momentum like a snowball
rolling downhill my progress got bigger and bigger
at the same time I let no one see me
so I trained in the gym covered with sweats
while Robbie trained in the gym shredded in rags
and won the contest everyday there at Gold's
but when it really counted he came to the contest
20 percent off his best
as he was losing, I was gaining
in the time remaining made sure
not to let negative thoughts enter my thinking
for I'd discovered a mantra and kept saying it all day
crowding out any negative thinking, thought only about
improving, it was not about anyone else but me.
Remember standing on stage that night October 1, 1977
with the top six I asked the universe to give me a sign
indicating I'd won so I could act more like the winner
and right at that time the head judge Oscar State
walked in front holding the list of the winners
and I saw my name in first place, it felt great!

DREAM LIFE

Life is a dream
life is real
a dream is a dream
a dream is real
when you're having it
when you're not
it's just a dream.
Life is real when you're living it
what about when you're not?

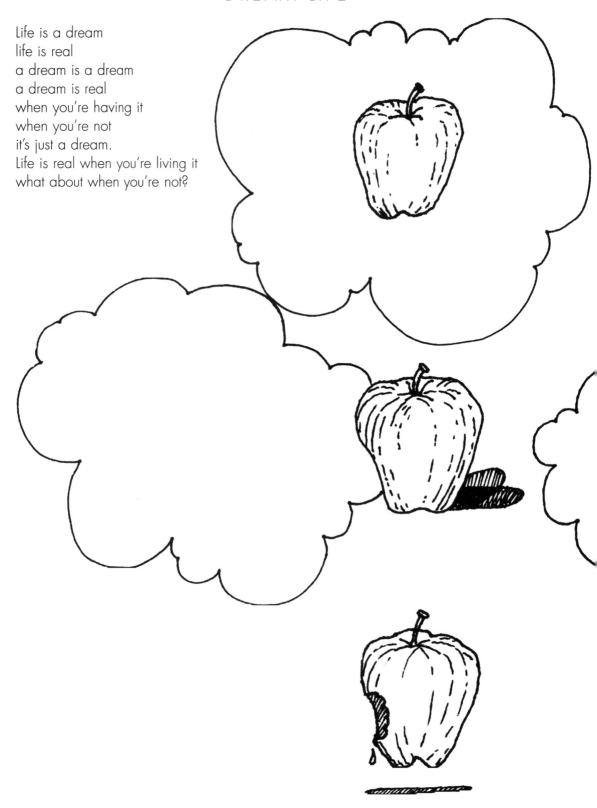

WORKOUT 89

Over 20 years ago here's the *back-chest-triceps* workout I did on a Friday, July 23, 1976, in preparation for the Mr. Olympia contest:

BACK
bent over barbell row
100, 120, 140, 150, and 160 pounds of 10 reps each
one-arm dumbbell row
80, 90, 95, and 100 pounds for 10 reps
front pulldown
170, 180, 190, and 200 pounds for 10 reps

CHEST (Dave Draper joining me for this tri-set)
{
dumbbell flys
55, 60, 65 pounds for 10 reps
cable flys
30, 35, and 40 pounds for three sets of 10 reps
dumbbell pullover
85 pounds for three sets of 10 reps
45 degree incline press on Smith machine
165, 185, and 195 pounds for 10 reps

TRICEPS
close grip bench press
135, 155, and 175 pounds for 10 reps (hands one foot apart)
lying triceps extension
85 pounds for 12 reps, 95 for 12, 105 for eight
one-arm dumbbell extension
35, 40, and 45 pounds for 10 reps
pressdown
four sets with 80 pounds
reverse dips
four sets of 10 reps with no weight

ABS
Roman chair situps
300 reps
incline knee in
two sets of 50 reps
crunches
100 reps straight out
hyperextension for spinal erectors
25 reps with 35 pounds
hung upside down with gravity boots (and rowing)
35 pounds for 10 reps

ran a mile in a lot by the gym

WORKOUT 90

The morning of July 24 in 1976 I trained *calves-thighs-abs* at Gold's Gym:

leg press
150 pounds for 20 reps, 170 for 16, 190 for 12
squatted
10 reps with 135, 185, 225, and 245 pounds
leg curl
10 reps with 60, 70, 80, and 90 pounds
leg extension
140 pounds for 12 reps, 160 for 10, 180 for 10, 200 for 10

CALVES
donkey calf raises
six sets of 25 reps with 30 seconds rest between sets (the 250-pound gym manager obligingly sat on my back, having big calves himself he understood the need for a heavy rider)
one-leg calf raise
four nonstop sets of 15 reps with no weight
seated calf machine
three sets of 15 reps

ABS
Roman chair situp
300 reps
leg raises
two sets of 40 reps
crunches
two sets of 60 reps
hyperextensions
with 10-pound plate for 20 reps

hung upside down five minutes holding a 50-pound weight doing 15 reps of rowing with it in this position; then let it drop to the floor and continued to hang for spinal traction

TRIP TO RHEO'S

Next day took a trip to Rheo's
almost like going to church for nourishment
picked up supplements, started with 15 to 20 aminos
per day and new enzymes three with each meal I'd take
didn't worry about fats in those days
watched only carbohydrate intake.
Rheo showed me a new way to eat eggs
first boil water, drop in egg for two minutes
crack shell drop in tall thin glass
pour in two ounces of beer
swallow with a few digestive enzyme pills
gained a few pounds of muscular bodyweight
from this it was clear.

WORKOUT 91

The cat woke me up early the next day in 1976. I ate a baked potato, slice of avocado, two eggs the Rheo way, sipped a few ounces of a protein drink, and got to the gym by 6:20 A.M.. The only one there before me was the Chief who said "you're late." After the following *delts-biceps-forearms* workout, I ran a mile so as not to feel guilty about skipping abs since my delts and elbows were sore and throbbing with pain; later I went to see Dr. Hexberg, my chiropractor. After he adjusted my neck and back, the pain was no longer a factor.

DELTS
dumbbell press
  10 reps with 50, 60, and 70 pounds
dumbbell seated upright row
  three sets of 10 reps with 50 pounds
overhead press machine
  135 pounds for 10 reps, 145 for 10, 160 for eight
one dumbbell front raise
  40, 45, and 50 pounds for 10 reps
dumbbell bent over rear delt raise
  20 pounds for 15 reps, 25 for 12, 30 for 10 (despite a
  pain in right rear delt and elbow, I didn't slow down)

BICEPS
alternate dumbbell curl
  with 35, 40, 45, and 50 pounders for eight to 12 reps
one-arm dumbbell concentration curl
  35, 40, 45, and 50 pounds between eight to 12 reps
preacher bench curl
  two sets of 12 reps with 50 pound barbell (a dull pain
  in my elbows began hurting like hell)

FOREARMS
{ **wrist curl with barbell**
  four sets of 20 reps with 75 pounds
reverse curl with barbell
  four sets of 10 reps with 65 pounds

TRAINING INSPIRATION IN 1976

Three things inspired me in training
for the Olympia in 1976:
the first was my low placing
in Mr. Olympia 1975 in South Africa
while "Pumping Iron" film was being made.
That year I got in shape two weeks too late
After the show did an exhibition in Berlin
West Germany looked great
for two days then drank wine and ate
candy didn't care, went to Paris, walked the streets
with Christine in November
it was really cold, felt bored
so went home to Santa Monica. I remember
saw Olympia on TV, wasn't even in it
then saw "Pumping Iron" movie, wasn't in that either
angry, embarrassed, went bowling, took it out on the pins
resolved that next year I would win.
Reason two, saw "Rocky" starring Sylvester Stallone
inspired me tremendously, he was then unknown.
Then in February 1976 did exhibition with Arnold and Ed Corney
at the Whitney Museum in New York City
not really in shape, had only been training two weeks
but the seeds of inspiration had been planted
gradually began training, getting ready, planning
to be in my greatest shape that year.
That summer of 1976, every night on TV in July
watched the summer Olympics from Montreal Canada
reason three, why I got so inspired, fired up for training
couldn't wait to go to the gym each day, kept gaining
size, strength, muscularity, resolved to improve my back
did eight sets bent over rowing at least three days a week
and by Olympia time had great lats
and spinal erectors like thick ropes, and delts and arms, too
and abs and legs and everything was in shape
still didn't win, got second place
missed by half a point, by sound of the applause
felt everybody in the joint that night in Columbus
thought I should have won, later analyzed mistakes I made
looking at photographs, saw a stoic expression always on my face.
Made up for it in 1977 Olympia, posed looking confident
and finally won first place.

WORKOUT 92

Woke up 5 A.M. on August 13, 1976, remembering a fragment from a dream about going up in an elevator. It's too crowded so I get out and take the next elevator by myself get to the top on my own. I eat breakfast and by 7 A.M., an hour later, I'm in the gym to work *back-chest-triceps-abs*. That night I had a dream which said keep on track, and in which I saw Franco Columbu walking around shirt off with a thick back.

BACK
bent over row
100, 120, 140, and 160 pounds for 10 reps
T bar row
100, 110, 120, and 130 pounds for 10 reps
one-arm dumbbell row
85, 100, and 110 pounds for 10 reps
close grip pulldown
three sets of 10 reps with 130 pounds
front pulldown
180, 190, and 200 pounds for eight reps
dumbbell pullover
80, 90, and 100 pounds for 10 reps

CHEST
dumbbell fly
55, 60, and 65 pounds for 10 reps
close grip bench press
135 pounds for 12 reps, 185 for 10, 225 for six

TRICEPS
one-arm dumbbell extension
35, 40, and 45 pounds for eight reps
reverse dips
15, 12, and 10 reps with 45-pound plate and only 30 seconds rest between sets
two-arm cable extension
three sets of 10 reps at 85 pounds

ABS
Roman chair situps
100 reps
hanging knee-ups
four sets of 25 reps
hyperextension
with hands behind head, no weight for 30 reps

WORKOUT 93

August 21, 1976 began *leg* workout.

leg press
15 reps with 150, 175, and 200 pounds
squatted
145, 165, 185, 205, and 235 pounds for 10 reps
leg curl
three sets of 10 reps with 80 pounds
leg extension
three sets of 10 reps with 180 pounds
donkey calf raise
(with Dave Draper on my back) six sets of 25 reps
leg press calf raise
four sets of 15 to 20 reps (stopped adding weight after 300 pounds)
hanging knee up
four sets of 30 reps with five-pound ankle weights on feet
hyperextension
30 reps with no weight

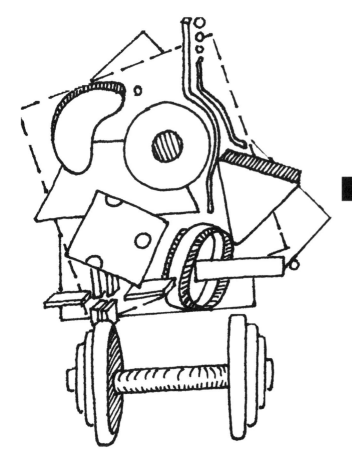

THOSE DAYS

Late 1970s to early 1980s
those compulsive training days
when I went to the gym every day
what else did we have to do anyway
that was more important than train?
But today
it's not exactly that way
as goals change with age
I realize there's so much
more to fill my day.
These days I feel blessed
by a day of rest.

WORKOUT 94

On August 23, 1976, I was in the gym by 6:50 A.M. to work on *delts-biceps-fore-arms*.

DELTS
dumbbell seated upright row
12 reps with 45, 50, and 55 pounds
rear delt cable raise
four sets with 20 pounds 10 reps
dumbbell press
70 pounds for 10 reps, 80 for 10, 90 for nine
machine press
145, 160, and 175 pounds for eight reps
dumbbell side raise
25, 30, and 35 pounds for 10 reps
one dumbbell front raise
50, 55, and 60 pounds
side cable raises
three nonstop sets with 15 pounds for 10 reps
wide grip front chin-ups
five sets of 10 reps

BICEPS
alternate dumbbell curl
40 pounds for 10 reps, 45 for nine, 50 for eight
incline dumbbell curl
three sets with 40 pounds for eight reps
dumbbell triceps kickback
three sets with 30 pounds for 10 reps
dumbbell concentration curl
35, 40, and 45 pounds for eight reps
preacher bench curl
three sets of 10 reps with 70 pounds

FOREARMS
reverse barbell curl
three sets of 10 reps with 85 pounds
wrist curl
85 pounds for three sets of 20 reps

I then drove up 4th Street to the 160 steps that climbed the side of Santa Monica canyon to the top. The first time ran them in 35 seconds and second time 45 seconds. Exhausted, I laid down at the top looking at the ocean then drove back to the gym where I worked on abs:

Roman chair situps
for 10 minutes (while talking to Ken Waller at 237 pounds looking pretty muscular but I wondered what his abs looked like that day)
hanging knee-ups
with ankle weights, four sets for 25 reps (while talking to Danny Padilla, another competitor, we were all friends in those days anyway)

MY 1978 WORKOUTS

Searching through my 1978 diary
reliving those workouts
can hardly believe it was me
who did all that stuff
that now seems way more than enough.

Can't help thinking no simplicity
here there's no parsimony.
Is this what I would still do
to win Mr. Olympia number two?

WORKOUT 95

At noon on August 21 in 1978, I trained *chest-lats-triceps-delts*:

CHEST
bench press
135 pounds for 15 reps, 185 for 10, 225 for 10, 245 for six
30-degree incline dumbbell press
80 pounds for 10 reps, 85 for 9, 90 for eight
decline fly
three sets of 10 reps with 55 pounds
pullover across flat bench with dumbbell
three sets of 10 reps with 90 pounds

LATS
one-arm dumbbell rowing
95 pounds for three set of 10
wide grip front chin
three sets of 10 reps

TRICEPS
pressdown
80 pounds for 10 reps, 90 for eight, 100 for seven
lying triceps extension
80 pounds for 10 reps, 90 for eight, 95 pounds for seven
one-arm dumbbell extension
35 pounds for 10 reps, 40 for eight, 45 for six
close grip bench press
(on the Smith machine)
three sets of eight reps with 185 pounds
dumbbell kickbacks
three sets of 10 reps with 30 pounders

I went home and returned to the gym at 4 P.M..

DELTS
dumbbell press
10 reps with 60, 65, and 70 pounds
seated dumbbell upright row
10 reps with 45, 50, and 55 pounds
bent over dumbbell rear delt raises
30 pounds for three sets of 10 reps

ABS
{ **hanging knee-ups**
{ **Roman chair situps**
both four sets of 25 reps

MONSTER DREAM

In a dream I'm being pursued
by a large monster man
not feeling any fear instead I use
my wits and rely on a plan
training for definition to subdue
these big 250-pound bodybuilders
let them win this year? Never!
I resolve to continue training harder than ever.

JULY 22

WORKOUT 96

At noon on August 22, 1978, I begin this great *back-biceps-forearms* workout:

front pulldown
 180, 190, 200, and 210 pounds for 10 reps
barbell bent over row
 100 pounds for 12 reps, 120 for 12, 140 for 12, 160 for 10, 170 for 10
one-arm dumbbell row
 100, 105, and 110 pounds for 10 reps
pulldown behind neck
 180, 200, 210, and 220 pounds for 10 reps (I used weight lifting straps so weight wouldn't slip)
barbell row (hanging upside down)
 60, 70, and 80 pounds for 10 reps
stiff arm pulldown
 80 pounds three sets of 10 reps

 BICEPS
alternate dumbbell curls
 40 pounds for 10 reps, 45 for 10, 50 for nine
barbell curl
 100, 110, and 120 pounds for eight to 10 reps
dumbbell incline curl
 40, 45, and 50 pounds for eight to 10 reps
preacher cable curl
 80, 90, and 100 pounds for 10 reps
one-arm concentration curl
 30, 35, and 40 pounds for 10 reps

 FOREARMS
barbell reverse curl
 80 pounds for four sets of 10 reps
barbell wrist curl
 four sets of 15 reps with 100-pound Olympic bar

WORKOUT 97

That same day of August 22, 1978, I was back in the gym at 6 P.M. to work on *thighs*:

leg press
150, 175, 200, and 225 pounds for 15 reps
leg extension
10 reps with 160, 180, and 190 pounds
leg curl
10 reps with 70, 80, and 90 pounds
standing one-leg curl
three sets of 10 with 35 pounds

CALVES
donkeys
(with a 210-pound rider) and holding a 50-pound
plate, five sets of 15 to 20 reps
leg press calf raise
four sets of 15 reps with 175 pounds
{ **hanging knee-up**
crunches
both for five sets of 25 reps

WORKOUT 98

On August 23, 1978, I began my morning with a *chest-triceps* workout.

bench press
135 pounds for 15 reps, 185 for 10, 225 for 10, 245 for nine, 265 for six
45-degree incline dumbbell press
80 pounds for 10, 90 pounds for eight, 100 pounds for six
decline fly
55 pound dumbbells three sets of 10
100 pound dumbbell pullover
three sets of 10 again
close grip bench press
three sets of 10 reps with 185 pounds
one-arm dumbbell extension
35 pounds for 10 reps, 40 for eight, 45 for seven
pressdown
three sets of 10 reps with 85 pounds
dumbbell kickback
30 pounds for three sets of 12 reps

I went home and ate a high-protein lunch and laid in the sun. Returned to the gym at 4 P.M. to work on *delts* and *abs*.

dumbbell press
60, 65, and 70 pounds for 10 reps
one dumbbell front raise
60, 65, and 70 pounds for 10 reps
seated dumbbell upright row
45 pounds for 12 reps, 50 for 10, 55 for nine
dumbbell side raise
four sets of 10 reps with only 20 seconds between sets
doing a pyramid
which means working up, then down in weight with 30, 35, 35, and 30 pounds

bent over rear delt raises
three sets with 30 pounds for 10 reps
one-arm cable row
three sets of 10 reps with 100 pounds

ABS
{ **hanging knee-up**
Roman chair situp
both four sets of 25 reps
hyperextension
25 reps
seated twists
100 reps

I walked down to the beach and ran along the shoreline barefoot in the wet sand for 10 minutes.

THIGH DEFINITION

My goal for winning Mr. Olympia 1978 was to have more definition
than in 1977 at the same bodyweight 187 and
get more striations in my quadriceps
so I purchased a Nautilus leg curl and leg extension
and installed them in my weekend suntanning house in Palm Springs
and after training all week in Santa Monica
concentrating mainly on upper body
in Palm Springs I'd do lots of sets of leg extension
leg curl & at the '78 Olympia had thigh cuts everybody could see easily.

WORKOUT 99

My second attempt to win the Mr. Olympia competition for a fourth time made me pursue a course of training which forced my body weight up to 209 pounds. I ate a lot of red meat and drank red wine because I've been told all my life "you need to get bigger." Though I took lots of time to build up my weight and trained five months for this contest, I came in second because I was too heavy. I competed almost injury free, but if I had to do it again I'd be five pounds lighter. Picking up my training from July 5, 1982 for *back-biceps-forearms*, here's what I did from 2 to 4 pm at World Gym:

BACK
dumbbell upright row
45 pounds for 12 reps, 50 for 12, 55 for 11, 60 for 10
low cable row
180, 200, 210, and 220 pounds for 10 reps
T bar row
115, 135, and 145 pounds for 10 reps
one-arm dumbbell row
110, 115, and 120 pounds for 10 reps
front pulldown
210 pounds for 10 reps, 220 for nine, 230 for eight, 240 for eight
close grip pulldown
160 pounds for 10 reps, 170 for nine, 180 for 10
hyperextension
holding a 25-pound plate for 20 reps

BICEPS
preacher cable curl
90 pounds for 10 reps, 100 for eight, 110 for seven
alternate dumbbell curl
40 pounds for 10 reps, 45 for nine, 50 for eight, 55 for seven
low incline dumbbell curl
30 pounds for 10 reps, 35 for nine, 40 for eight

FOREARMS
barbell reverse curl
three sets of 10 reps with 90 pounds
wrist curl
three sets of 20 reps with 100 pounds

ABS
Roman chair situps
200 reps
hanging knee-ups
four sets of 25 reps
seated twists
100 reps

Later I walked two miles, then ate supper.

WORKOUT 100

Began working calves the next day:

one-legged raise
each leg, holding a 25-pound weight, three sets of 15 reps
seated calf raise machine
three sets with 110 pounds for 15 reps
donkey calf raise
three sets with 220 pounds for 18 reps

THIGHS
leg curl
90 pounds for 12 reps, 95 for 11, 100 for 10
lunges
10 reps at 60, 70, and 80 pounds
leg extension
10 reps at 140, 160, and 180 pounds
front squat
10 reps at 100, 110, and 120 pounds

ABS
{**incline leg raise**
four sets of 30 reps
crunches
holding 10 pounds, four sets of 30 reps

one-arm cable crunch
two sets of 25 reps for each arm with 70 pounds

I ended the workout with a 14-minute walk outside.

WORKOUT 101

On July 7 in 1982 I trained *chest-triceps-delts* at the World Gym from 7 to 8:30 A.M..

75-degree incline dumbbell front press
50 pounds for 12 reps, 60 for 11, 70 for 10 reps
30-degree incline press on Smith machine
155 pounds for 10 reps, 175 for nine, 195 for eight

LOWER PECS
dumbbell fly
45, 50, and 55 pounds for 10 reps
dumbbell pullover
70, 80, and 90 pounds for 10 reps

TRICEPS
close grip bench press
135 pounds for 10 reps, 155 for eight, 175 for six
one-arm dumbbell extension
35 pounds for 10 reps, 40 for eight, 45 for seven
pressdown
80 pounds for 10 reps, 85 for nine, 90 for eight
dumbbell kickback
30 pounds for 12 reps, 35 for 11, 40 for 10

DELTS
press behind neck on the Smith machine
75, 80, and 90 pounds for 10 reps
bent over dumbbell rear delt raises
three sets of 10 reps with 30 pounds
dumbbell side raises
25, 30, and 35 pounds for 10 reps
one-arm side cable raises
20 pounds three sets of 10 reps each arm nonstop

I went home, ran for 10 minutes in the park, relaxed, ate, took a nap, awoke, had some black coffee, then returned to the gym at 3 P.M. where I did *abs*:

{ **Roman chair situp**
five sets of 30 reps
leg raises
five sets of 30 reps
{ **hanging knee-ups**
seated twist
both for two sets of 50 reps
hyperextension
20, 15, and 15 reps with 25 pounds

THE 5-4-5 SEQUENCE

In the past I used a four-day sequence to get into top shape
which means I'd train three days in a row then rest one day
working each body part once in four days and abs all three workout days
and a total of two hours a week of aerobics at the end of each workout to
get in peak shape
but found after a month of four-day sequence I was getting overtrained.
There's a way to avoid this and build size, strength and definition.
It's the 5-4-5 sequence and it means training the whole body in five days
then four then five again and it will start all over again after two weeks.
Another benefit is you will always have the same day off every week.
Here it is using a three-way split: on, on, off, on, off (five days) then
on, on, on, off (four days) then on, on, off, on, off (five days) and begin again.

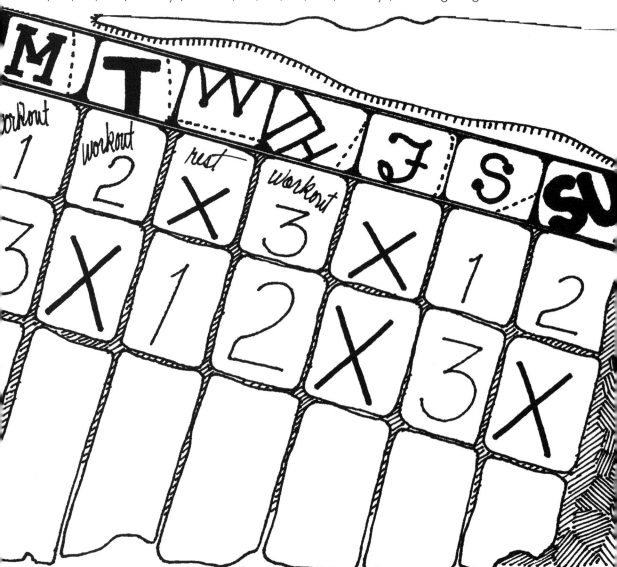

W O R K O U T 1 0 2

When doing this back-biceps-forearms workout of mine from July 1982 keep in mind that the weights are relative—don't try to use the same weights, sets, and reps as I did. I just want to show the training I did over the years to get into top shape:

BACK
two-arm lat stretch
low cable row
  160, 180, 200, and 220 pounds for 10 reps
T bar row (leverage row)
  with 125 pounds for 10 reps, 150 for nine, 160 for eight
one-arm dumbbell row
  115 pounds for 10 reps, 120 for 10, 125 for eight
dumbbell upright row
  45 pounds for 12 reps, 50 for 11, 55 for 10
front pulldown
  200, 210, 220, 230, and 240 pounds for 10 reps
close grip pulldown
  170, 180, 190, and 200 pounds for 10 reps

BICEPS
preacher cable curl
  60 and 70 pounds for 10 reps, and 80 for eight
alternate dumbbell curl
  45 pounds for 10 reps, 50 for nine, 55 for eight, 60 for six
incline dumbbell curl
  35 and 40 pounds for 10 reps, 45 for eight
one-arm dumbbell concentration curl
  45 pounds for eight reps, 50 for seven, 55 for six

I drove home, ran for 10 minutes, ate, relaxed, recuperated a little, and was back in the gym by 3:30 P.M..

FOREARMS
barbell reverse curl
  80, 90, and 100 pounds for 10 reps
barbell wrist curl
  80, 90, and 100 pounds for 15 reps

ABS
{ **hanging knee-ups**
 crunches
   both three sets of 40 reps
{ **Roman chair situp**
 incline leg raise
   both four sets of 25 reps
seated twist
  100 reps
hyperextension
  two sets of 15 reps

WORKOUT 103

The next day I drove to Palm Springs. It was 112 degrees outside, so I stayed inside with the air conditioning and began *calves* and *abs* training at 5:15 P.M. at my Zane Haven gym.

calf raise drop sets with the Leg Blaster
180 pounds for 20 reps, drop to 140 for 12, stretch and rest three minutes
200 pounds for 16 reps, drop to 160 for 12, rest and stretch again
220 pounds for 15 reps, drop to 180 for 10, rest a little longer

seated calf raise
120, 110, and 100 pounds for 12 reps each, resting only 30 seconds between sets

leg curl
three sets of 12 reps with 90 pounds

leg extension
three sets of 15 reps with 150 pounds

ABS

crunches
50 reps, (holding a three-pound dumbbell on my chest)

incline leg raise
50 reps

seated twist
100 reps

hyperextensions
25 reps

When I went outside, it seemed like a sauna, so I dove into my pool and swam four laps.

BILL PEARL

One bodybuilding contest I think of still
is the 1971 Professional Mr. Universe in London
where I competed against Bill Pearl.
I learned that the real secret to winning is
act like the winner before you win.
After spending the summer doing exhibitions
and seminars in South Africa and the rest of
the time doing nothing but training
sometimes six hours a day
getting ready to compete with Pearl and Sergio Oliva
knew Arnold wouldn't be there
he was already Mr. Olympia.
Weighing 194 with razor sharp definition I flew to London.
Won my class division easily in prejudging then
readied myself for a head on confrontation with the other class winner
which never came. Felt it was really lame the judges didn't compare
all the winners. Watching Pearl show exactly what he wanted everyone
to see, it was obvious to me that he knew exactly what to do.
It was his last competition which he won at age 41.
This was not the only thing I learned from a legend
with the same name as my birthstone
Pearl one of a kind.

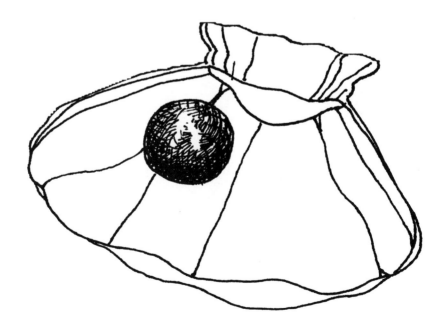

WORKOUT 104

Next day I did a *chest-triceps-delts* workout. Afterwards at 9 P.M., I ran and walked a mile.

CHEST
75-degree incline dumbbell press
55 pounds for 15 reps, 65 for 12, 75 for 10
30-degree incline barbell press
140 pounds for 10 reps, 170 for nine, 190 for eight with slow negatives
dumbbell fly
50 pounds for 10 reps, 55 for 10, 60 for 10
dumbbell pullover
75 pounds for 12 reps, 85 for 11, 95 for 10

TRICEPS
close grip bench press
140 pounds for 10 reps, 170 for eight, 190 for six
one-arm dumbbell extension
35 pounds for 12 reps, 45 for 10, 50 for eight
pressdown
three sets of 10 reps with 80 pounds
kickback
30 pounds for 12 reps, 35 for 11, 40 for 10

I rested, ate, and lay out in the sun before returning to my workout at 4:45 P.M..

DELTS
press behind neck
90 pounds for 11 reps, 100 for 10, 110 for nine
dumbbell side raise
30, 35, and 40 pounds for 10 reps
bent over dumbbell rear delt raises
25, 30, and 35 pounds for 10 reps
rear delt cable raises
three sets of 10 reps with 20 pounds
one-arm side cable raise
three sets of 10 reps with 30 pounds nonstop and alternating arms

ABS
pulley knee-in
45 pounds for four sets of 25 reps
{ **incline leg raise**
crunches
both five pounds for 30 reps
one-arm 85-pound cable crunch
four sets of 25

PROTEIN, CARBOHYDRATE, AND FAT

How much protein, carbohydrate, and fat in my diet?
My opinion is that in normal training with weights
carbohydrate exceeds protein by one-third
eating at least one gram of protein per pound of body weight
this gives enough energy to
train hard and get a good pump.
But last month before competition the pendulum swung
the other way, that is to say weighing 180
eat 240 grams of protein and 180 grams of carbs
and don't eat starches late in the day.
Losing puffiness I'd drop excess water this way
and my fats would stay under 25 percent of my total calorie intake.

WORKOUT 105

At 6:30 A.M. on July 13 in 1982 I ran 12 minutes before it got hot, ate a breakfast of three soft boiled eggs and a small yam, sunbathed, then trained *back-biceps-forearms-abs* in my gym:

hyperextension
10 pounds for 15 reps, 25 for 10

top deadlift
(that is, deadlift from the knees up on my power rack after rubbing oil on my thighs to make the bar slide up easily; I used weight lifting straps with a grip that is slightly wider than the normal shoulder width)
235 pounds for 12 reps, 325 for 11, 415 for 10, 485 for eight

low cable row
180, 200 and 210 pounds for 10 reps, 220 for eight

one-arm dumbbell row
115 pounds for 10 reps, 120 for nine, 125 for eight

dumbbell upright row
50, 55, and 60 pounds for 10 reps

pulldown behind neck
190, 200, and 210 pounds for 10 reps

I then took a three-minute break.

{
front chin
three sets of 10 reps each
sideways swings
10 reps

close grip pulldown
160 and 170 pounds for 10 reps, 180 pounds for eight

dumbbell row (hanging by my feet upside down)
20 pounds for 15 reps, 30 for 12

BICEPS

preacher cable curl
65 pounds for 10 reps, 70 for nine, 80 for eight

dumbbell concentration curl
three sets of six reps at 40 pounds with only 20 seconds rest between sets

alternate dumbbell curl
45 pounds for nine reps, 50 for eight, 55 for seven

FOREARMS

{
reverse curl
90 and 100 pounds for 10 reps
wrist curl with barbell
70 pounds for 12 reps, 80 for 10

ABS

pulley knee-in
four sets of 25 reps at 50 pounds

{
incline knee-in
crunches
both five sets of 30 reps

one-arm cable crunches
two sets of 25 reps at 80 pounds with each arm

WORKOUT 106

Next day ran again for 12 minutes in the already hot morning. After breakfast I laid an hour in the sun, before beginning my *calves-thighs-abs* workout with some calf stretching.

standing calf raise drop sets
240 pounds for 20 reps, drop to 180 for 15; rest three minutes; 260 for 15, drop to 200 for 15; rest three minutes; 280 for 15, drop to 220 for 10

seated calf raise
100, 110, 115, and 120 pounds for 12 reps

one-legged calf raise
three sets of 15 reps holding a 35-pound dumbbell

thighs
leg curl, 80 pounds for 12 reps, 90 for 11, 100 for 10

lunges
10 reps with 60, 70, and 80 pounds

leg extension
160 pounds for 11 reps, 180 for 10, 200 for nine

front squat
100, 110, and 120 pounds for 10 reps

ABS
incline leg raise
five sets of 30 reps
crunches
five sets of 40 reps

OBLIQUES
one-arm cable crunches
two sets of 25 reps each arm with 85 pounds, followed by two sets of 25 reps with 95 pounds each arm

hyperextension
10 pounds for 15, 15, and 10 reps

AEROBICS

Next day sunbathed a few hours and rested well.
After the sun set and thermometer dropped to 95 degrees
walked a mile at Palm Springs High track in 16:36 minutes
then felt a breeze blowing on my back
so ran backward for a lap with my eyes
on the white line marking the lane I was in
so I didn't bump into anyone who
happened to be running there too.
Forward running and walking works frontal thighs
and tibialis, while running backward
hits the leg biceps, calves and lower back.
I really feel it in my butt when I lean a little forward.

WORKOUT 107

July 15th 7 to 8:15 A.M. I began my *chest-triceps* workout at my Zane Haven gym starting with

75-degree incline dumbbell press
60 pounds for 12 reps, 65 for 11, 70 for 10
30-degree incline barbell press
140 pounds for 10 reps, 170 for nine, 200 for eight, 210 pounds for six
dumbbell flyes
45 pounds for 12 reps, 50 for 11, 55 for 10
dumbbell pullover
80, 90, and 100 pounds for 10 reps

TRICEPS
close grip barbell bench press
140 and 170 pounds for 10 reps, 190 for eight
one-arm dumbbell extension
40 pounds for 10, 45 for nine, 50 for eight

pressdown
85 pounds for three sets of 10 reps
dumbbell kickbacks
30, 35, and 40 pounds for 10 reps

Then I drove to Santa Monica and was in the gym by 4:15 to work on *deltoids* and *abs*:

press behind neck on the Smith machine
75, 95, and 115 pounds for 10 reps
bent over rear delt raises with dumbbells
25, 30, and 35 pounds for 10 reps
dumbbell side raises
35, 40, and 45 pounds for 10 reps
one dumbbell front raise
65, 70, and 75 pounds for 10 reps
one-arm dumbbell side raises
20, 25, and 30 pounds for 10 reps
one-arm side cable raises
three nonstop sets with 20 pounds alternating each arm

{
hanging knee-up
Roman chair situp
both four sets of 30 reps
{
leg raise
crunches
both five sets of 30 reps
one-arm cable crunch
35 pounds for two sets of 25 reps with each arm

hyperextension
20 reps, then 10 pounds for 15 reps

PASSING OF TIME

Getting ready for London Mr. Olympia
late this year November 13, 1982
there was no time for poetry
just hard training.
I was in very good shape weighing over 200 pounds
with only two weeks remaining
my goal was to compete at this bodyweight
or very close to it, realize now this was a mistake
should have forgotten about the scale
and focused instead on muscular detail.

WORKOUT 108

I preceeded my *back-biceps-forearms* workout on October 28 in 1982 at 6:40 A.M. with an hour bike ride. After finishing at 11:30 A.M., I ate lunch, then went out by the pool to get two hours of sun to deepen my tan for London. A refreshing breeze blew through the palm trees making the 90 degrees actually feel cool.

BACK
top deadlift
235 pounds for 15 reps, 325 for 12, then 415, 485, and 535 for 10
low cable row
180, 200, and 210 pounds for 10 reps, 220 for eight
one-arm dumbbell row
105 pounds for 12 reps, 115 for 11, 125 for 10
front chin and sideways swing
three sets of 10 reps
close grip pulldown
150 pounds three sets of 10 reps
pulldown behind neck
180 pounds for 15 reps, 190 for 12, 200 for 10
one-arm cable row
100 pounds for 16 reps, 110 for 15, 120 for 12

BICEPS/FOREARMS
preacher cable curl
100 pounds for 15 reps, 110 for 12, 120 for 10

UPPER OUTER BICEPS
low incline dumbbell curl
30 pounds for 12 reps, 35 for 10, 40 for nine, 45 for eight

TOP OF FOREARMS AND LOWER BICEPS
{ **EZ bar reverse preacher curl**
70 pounds for 10 reps, 80 for 10, 90 for eight
barbell wrist curl
three sets of 90 pounds for 12 reps

ABS
pulley knee
60 pounds around my ankles for five sets of 20 reps
{ **hanging leg raise**
crunches
both four pounds for 25 reps
one-arm cable crunch
100 pounds two sets of 25 with each arm
seated twist
100 reps
hyperextension
three sets of 15 reps

WORKOUT 109

On November 4 in 1982 I started my *leg* workout at 7:45 A.M.. In those days before the Leg Blaster, I worked on my thighs by doing a full squat with a barbell on my upper back. I remember I had to grip the seven-foot Olympic bar all the way out to the side collars, which not only pumped up my thighs but worked on my biceps, neck, and shoulders.

CALVES
one leg calf raises
with 40-pound dumbbell in one hand while holding on for balance with the other, three sets of 15 reps each leg
donkeys
with a 200-pound rider, four sets of 25 reps
seated calf raise
100 pounds for 20 reps, 110 for 18, 120 for 16

THIGHS
squats
first set with 165-pounds for 20 reps followed by laying on the floor five minutes
second set with 215 pounds for 20 reps, again another floored performance
third set with 255 pounds for 20 reps, and another five minutes on the floor
leg curl
90 pounds for 12 reps, 100 for 11, 110 for 10
one-leg curl
50 pounds for three sets of 10 reps
leg extension
180 pounds for 15 reps, 200 for 13, 220 for 10
one-leg top extension
60 pounds 12, 10, and eight reps with each leg

After finishing at 10 A.M., ate lunch, went out by my pool and got two hours of sun. Then at 4 P.M. I rode my bike 50 minutes and at 6 P.M. did 20 minutes of ab stimulation on my electric impulse machine followed by regular *ab* work:

{ **incline leg raise**
crunches
both five sets of 30 reps
{ **one-arm cable crunch**
100 pounds for two sets of 25 reps each arm
seated twist
two sets of 50 reps
hyperextension
15 pounds for three sets of 15 reps

That night at 8 P.M. I used my electric machine on my lower back for 20 minutes at low current threshold for healing and improving circulation, then lay on an ice pack for 20 minutes numbing the pain in my rear delts and traps.

WORKOUT 110

My last *chest-shoulder-triceps* workout before the 1982 Mr. Olympia came on November 5 from 3:45 to 6 P.M. after sunning two hours.

75-degree incline dumbbell press
65 pounds for 12 reps, 70 for 10, 75 for nine, 80 for eight

25-degree incline barbell press
190 pounds for 10 reps, 210 for eight, 230 for six

bench press
210 pounds for 10 reps, 230 for eight, 250 for five, 270 for two, all with very slow negatives of up to 10 seconds

one-dumbbell front raise
70 pounds for 12 reps, 75 for 11, 80 for 10

dumbbell flyes
50 pounds for 15 reps, 60 for 12, 70 for eight

dumbbell pullover lying across the bench
95 pounds for 12 reps, 105 for 12, 115 for 10

one-arm dumbbell extension
35 pounds for 10 reps, 40 for 10, 45 for eight, 50 for six

pressdown
90 pounds for three sets of eight reps holding the lockout one second

dumbbell kickback
35 pounders for four sets of 15 reps

DELTS
side raise with dumbbells
40, 45, and 50 pounds for 12 reps

one-arm cable row
100, 110, and 120 pounds for 10 reps

I then lay on the floor and did 20 minutes with my electric machine: putting the pads on my lower abs while turning the current up higher and higher in order to force them to contract harder.

pulley knee-in
75 pounds for five sets of 20 reps

crunches
40, 30, and 30 reps

one-arm cable crunch
110 pounds for two sets of 25 reps with each arm

seated twists
100 reps

PHOTOS—
EVIDENCE OF MY BODYBUILDING CAREER

Remember two days later in Santa Monica
looking at photos Artie Zeller took of my training at Zane Haven
and posing in the desert with Mt. San Jacinto in the background
excellent they were and still are some of the best photos I've seen.
Later Sunday that day took photos with John Balik now owner of
Ironman magazine. Then for some reason I think of the "Plot of the Alien Dream."
Going back through time to January 1981 remember a dream; don't know what it means
I'm escaping an alien type force very bright, huge, smiling
awesome, descends on me different times and finds me each time
hiding in protection, then escape it in a rocket ship, with another person.
The rocket ship's in the shape of a metal bookcase and I squeezed into the top shelf
while the crew member squeezed into the bottom of the three shelves, maybe there's four
not more, a takeoff crew closes up the ship. We fire off.

WORKOUT 111

It's July 17, 1980, Christine and I have just returned from a week vacation in Puerta Vallarta, Mexico, after running the 1980 Zane Invitational Women's Bodybuilding tournament. It lost money, but we didn't care since we needed a vacation. I now find myself in the World Gym on Main Street in Santa Monica where I'm about to begin a two-hour workout at 8:30 A.M. on *back-biceps-forearms* with 11 weeks left before the 1980 Mr. Olympia in Sydney, Australia.

BACK
barbell rowing
130, 150, 170, and 190 pounds for 10 reps
top deadlift
225, 315, and 405 pounds for 10 reps, 475 for eight, 525 for four (I could have done more but my weight lifting straps slipped and I lost my grip.)
dumbbell shrug
90, 100, and 110 pounds for 10 reps
one-arm dumbbell row
95 pounds for three sets of 10 reps
pulldown behind neck
230, 250, and 270 pounds for 10 reps
low cable row
180 and 190 pounds for 10 reps

BICEPS
barbell curl
100 pounds for 10 reps, 110 for nine, 120 for eight, 130 for six
low incline dumbbell curl
35 and 40 pounds for 10 reps, 45 for eight, 50 for six
preacher cable curl
100 pounds for eight, 110 for seven, 110 for six, 110 for 6

FOREARMS
reverse barbell curl
65, 75, 85, and 95 pounds for 10 reps
wrist curl (on a five-foot Olympic bar)
four sets of 15 reps with 100 pounds

ABS
{ **Roman chair situp**
incline knee-in
both for 40, 30, and 30 reps
seated twist
100 reps
hyperextension
two sets of 20 reps

WORKOUT 112

Written on the brown pages of my leather-bound wood-covered book is the workout I did on July 19, 1980. Early the day before I drove to Palm Springs, ran one and a half miles at the local high school track, and weighed in at 204 pounds before bed. I woke the next morning feeling that I'm bigger and stronger as I got ready to work *legs* at my home gym—a little weekend workout, relaxation, and sunbathing house in which two of the three bedrooms were my gym. I recorded in the book that I ate only 100 grams of carbohydrate that day.

leg extension
160, 180, and 200 pounds for 10 reps
one-legged top extension
60 pounds for 15, 70 for 12, 80 for 10
squat on my power rack
145, 195, 235, 275, 305, and 330 pounds for 10 reps
lunges
90 and 100 pounds for 10 reps
leg curl
90, 100, and 110 pounds for 10 reps
stiff-legged deadlift
85, 95, and 105 pounds for 10 reps (to stretch the hamstrings)
hyperextension
three sets of 10 reps holding 10, then 20, then 30 pounds behind my head (for butt, spinal erectors, and upper hamstrings)
seated calf raise
110, 120, 130, and 140 pounds for 15 reps
donkeys
with 220 pounds on lower back, five sets of 20 to 25 reps

After sundown I ran a mile and a half in 15 minutes at the high school track then returned home to an *abs* workout:

{
crunches
hanging knee-ups
both four sets of 25 reps
seated twists
100 reps

WHAT I ATE

July 10, 1980 woke up had two cups of coffee
sweetened with aspartame and glycine
then I ate two tablespoons milk egg protein powder mixed with
12 ounces cottage cheese with one cup of fresh strawberries
For lunch, one papaya, 12 ounces chicken and a lite beer
Late afternoon, 16 ounces yogurt 12 cherries 16 pecans a few macadamia nuts
For dinner, 16 ounces chicken one piece of rye bread with
four ounces of cheese melted on it, then before bed had two eggs Rheo way
with another lite beer and three grams of L-tryptophan and went to sleep.

WORKOUT 113

On July 20, 1980 I did the following ***chest-shoulder-triceps-abs*** workout from 10:10 A.M. to 12:20 P.M. in Palm Springs:

CHEST
bench press
145 pounds for 20 reps, 195 for 12, 235 for 10, 260 for six, and four sets of one rep doing slow negative with 285 pounds
30-degree incline dumbbell press
70 and 75 pounds for 10 reps, 80 for nine, 85 for seven
V bar dips
(same as parallel dip but with a V-shaped bar) three sets of 15 reps
dumbbell pullover
three sets of 12 reps with 95 pounds

DELTS
75 degree incline dumbbell press
60 pounds for 10 reps, 65 for eight, 70 for five, 55 for seven
one dumbbell front raise
55, 65, and 70 pounds for 10 reps
dumbbell side raise
25, 30, and 35 pounds for 10 reps
rear delt cable raise (bent over at the waist)
15 pounds for four sets of 12 reps
one-arm side cable raise
20, 25, and 30 pounds 10 reps

TRICEPS
one-arm cable kickback
25, 30, and 35 pounds for 10 reps
close grip bench press
165 and 185 pounds for eight reps, 205 for seven
pressdown
70 pounds for 12 reps, 80 for 10, 90 for nine, 100 for eight
one-arm dumbbell extension
35 and 40 pounds for 10 reps, 45 for eight

ABS
pulley knee-in
35 pounds around my ankles for four sets of 25 reps
hanging knee up
four sets of 25 reps
crunches
four sets of 25 reps
hyperextension
two sets of 20 reps

1980 OLYMPIA OUTCOME
DISGUISED IN A DREAM

I have a job in a movie as an archer to shoot and hit
a vibrating two-inch diameter rubber circular target.
There I am going to job dressed in a clown suit
driving in the left hand turn lane when here comes a truck
carrying two elephants for the movie set
and makes a right turn before me.
I follow to the set and the director Wink Martindale
asks me how to play the part of a bodybuilder.
Christine and I suggest posing
and I wonder why I'm dressed like a clown.
Looking at two-inch archery target, the movie crew is vibrating
to give effect of arrow hitting it and I realize that
I don't have to shoot at it after all.

WORKOUT 114

Late morning on July 21, 1980 in Palm Springs, I trained **back-biceps-forearms-abs**. Later that evening, I ran a mile and a half in 15 minutes at the high school track.

bent over barbell rowing
150, 170, and 190 pounds for 10 reps

top deadlift
235, 325, and 415 pounds for 10 reps, 485 for eight, 535 for six (my straps slipped and I lost my grip on the bar)

dumbbell shrug
95 pounds for three sets of 10 reps

pulldown behind neck
230, 240, and 250 pounds for 12 reps

one-arm dumbbell row
three sets of 10 reps with 95 pounds

low cable row
170 pounds for 10 reps, 180 for nine, 190 for eight

one-arm cable row
two sets of 10 reps with 100 pounds

BICEPS
barbell curl
100 pounds for 10 reps, 110 for nine, 120 for eight, 130 for seven, 140 for six (put rubbing liniment on my elbows)

incline dumbbell curl
40, 45, 45, and 50 pounds for 8 reps

one-arm dumbbell concentration curl
three sets of eight reps with 40 pounds

FOREARMS
reverse preacher bench curl with EZ curl bar
65 pounds for 10 reps, 70 for eight, 75 for seven

barbell reverse curl
80, 90, and 100 pounds for 10 reps

wrist curl
90 pounds for 15 reps, 80 for 12

ABS
pulley knee-in
40 pounds for four sets of 25 reps

{ **hanging knee-ups**
crunches
both four sets of 25 reps

hyperextension
10 pounds for 20 reps, 20 for 12, 30 for 10

WORKOUT 115

Two days later at 9:30 A.M. I worked on *legs* in the World Gym.

squats
185, 225, 275, 315, 335, and 355 pounds for 10 reps
standing calf raise
200, 220, and 240 pounds for 15 reps
seated calf raise
100, 110, 120, and 130 pounds for 15 reps
incline calf raises face down on hack machine
200 pounds for three sets of 15 reps

After driving to a Santa Monica Nautilus center:

leg extension
150, 160, and 170 pounds for 12 reps
leg curl
90, 100, and 110 pounds for 10 reps

ABS
incline knee-in
two sets of 50 reps
hanging knee-up
three sets of 40, 30, and 30 reps
hyperextension
20 reps

At the end of the day, feeling that my L-5 vertebrae was out, I spent an hour in the hot tub, then drove to Palm Spring with ice on lower back for two hours.

WORKOUT 116

Next day at my home gym in Palm Springs, I worked *chest-delts-triceps* from 11 A.M. to one P.M..

bench press
145 pounds for 15 reps, 210 for 10, 245 for six, 255 for six, 265 for five, 270 for five, 275 for four, slow negatives on all sets

incline dumbbell press
70 pounds for 10 reps, 80 for eight, 85 for six

V bar dip
three sets of 15 reps with 20 pounds around my waist

decline dumbbell fly
60 pounds for three sets of 10 reps

dumbbell pullover
three sets of 95 pounds for 10 reps

high incline dumbbell press
60 pounds for 10 reps, 65 for eight, 70 for eight, 75 for six

one dumbbell front raise
55, 65, and 70 pounds for 10 reps

dumbbell side raise
25 and 30 pounds for 10 reps, 35 for eight

dumbbell rear delt raise (face down on steep incline bench)
25 pounds for three sets of 10 reps

bent over rear cable raise
three sets of 20 pounds for 10 reps

one-arm side cable raise
three sets of 5 reps with 25 pounds

TRICEPS
dumbbell kickback
25 pounds for 15 reps, 30 for 12, 35 for 10

close grip bench press (with elbows out)
195 pounds for eight reps, 205 for seven, 215 for five—20 seconds rest—215 for four

pressdown
70 and 80 pounds for 10 reps, 90 for eight, 100 pounds for six

one-arm dumbbell extension
35 and 40 pounds for 10 reps, 45 for eight

hanging knee-ups
four sets of 25 reps

I ate lunch, lay in the sun for an hour, took a two and half hour nap, got up and had a snack, then from 10 to 10:30 P.M.:

donkey calf raises
240 pounds for 25, 25, 25, 20, and 20 reps

pulley knee-in
35 pounds four sets of 25 reps

stairclimber
five minutes

FOOD I ATE

That day I ate a total of 16 ounces cottage cheese, two cups of string beans
10 ounces of steak, 16 more ounces cottage cheese, milk and egg protein
mixed in with 16 ounces yogurt with two peaches
thinking about it today this is way too much whey protein
totaling 240 grams protein, 180 grams carb, 3700 calories
drank a half bottle of Zinfandel spread throughout latter part of the day
came in handy when I wanted to sleep easily
and numb lower back pain still persisting from yesterday
later lay on ice pack for half an hour before bed.

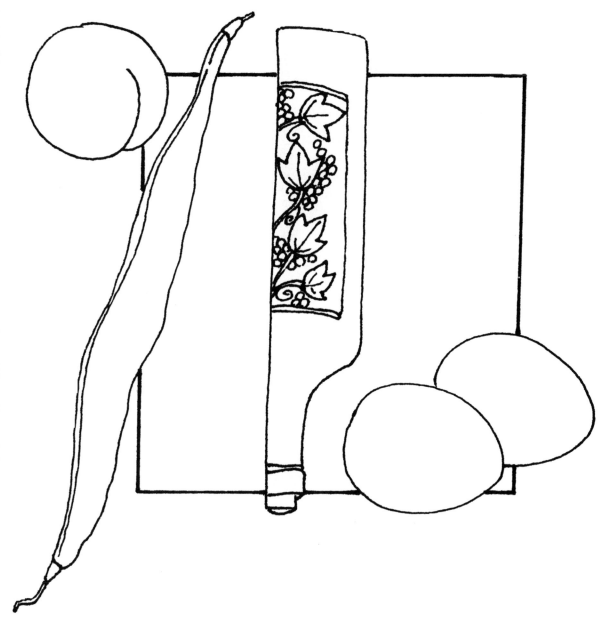

WORKOUT 117

Next workout in Palm Springs came a few days later at 10 A.M. in my home gym:

BACK

top deadlift
235, 325, and 415 pounds for 10 reps, 465 for eight, 505 for three reps
I lost my grip on the fourth repetition because my weight lifting straps slipped and I dropped the weight. Cursing my fate shrugged ahead:

dumbbell shrugs
95 pounds for three sets of 10 reps (compared to deadlift, shrugging was easy)

pulldown behind neck
230 pounds for 10 reps, 240 pounds for 10, 250 pounds for 10

front pulldown
190 pounds for 10 reps, 200 pounds for 10, 210 pounds for eight; on the ninth rep I forgot if I was doing pulldown to front or behind the neck and pulled the bar straight down hard on my head; seeing stars and bleeding, I said "What the hell is wrong with me," as I iced my bruise and did instead:

one-arm dumbbell row
95 pounds two sets of 10 reps

low cable row
180 pounds for 10 reps, 190 for nine, 200 for eight

one-arm cable row
two sets of 10 reps with 110 pounds

BICEPS

dumbbell concentration curl
four sets of eight reps with a 40-pound dumbbell

preacher cable curl
80, 90, and 100 pounds for 10 reps

low incline curl
35 pounds for 10 reps, 40 for eight, and 40 for seven

FOREARMS

EZ bar reverse preacher curl
three sets of eight reps with 65 pounds

reverse curl
85, 95, and 105 pounds for 10 reps

barbell wrist curl
80 pounds for 15 reps, 90 for 12

I rested a while and had all but forgotten about the bruise on my head.

pulley knee-in (around my ankles)
45 pounds for four sets of 25 reps

crunches
two sets of 50 reps

hyperextensions
20 reps

treadmill
15 minutes

WORKOUT 118

Worked *legs* the next day at 10:15 A.M.:

THIGHS
one-leg top extension
60, 70, and 80 pounds for 15 reps
squatting
145, 195, 235, 275, 305, and 325 pounds for 10 reps
leg extension
160, 170, and 180 pounds for 10 reps
lunge
80 and 90 pounds for 10 reps
leg curl
three sets of 10 reps with 100 pounds
stiff legged deadlift
three sets of 10 reps with 70 pounds

CALVES
seated calf raises
110, 120, and 130 pounds for 15 reps
donkeys (with 230-pound rider)
four sets for 15 reps

LOWER BACK
hyperextension
four sets of 10 reps

ABS
hanging knee-ups
four sets of 25 reps
pulley knee-in
40 pounds for four sets of 25 reps
stairclimber
12 minutes

WORKOUT 119

Following an hour of sun, I began a ***chest-shoulders-triceps-abs*** workout at 11:30 A.M.. Afterwards my front delts were really sore, so I did electric current then put on a tight T-shirt and slipped a blue ice strip in for 30 minutes and took a few buffered aspirin.

bench press
145 pounds for 14 reps, 215 for 10, 255 for five, then 260, 265, 270, and 275 for six all with slow negatives
incline dumbbell press
75 pounds for eight reps, 80 for seven, 85 for six, all slow negatives
V bar dips
with 25 pounds around my waist, three sets of 16 reps
decline dumbbell fly
60 pounds for two sets of 10 reps
dumbbell pullover
three sets of 10 reps with 95 pounds

DELTS
dumbbell press (at 75 degrees incline)
60 pounds for 10 reps, 70 for nine, 75 for eight
one dumbbell front raise
60, 70, and 70 pounds for 10 reps
dumbbell side raise
30 pounds for 12 reps, 35 for 10, 40 for eight
rear delt raise
(face down on steep incline bench)
25 pounds for three sets of 10 reps
bent over rear delt cable raise
four sets of 10 reps with 20 pounds
one-arm side cable raise
two sets of 10 reps with 30 pounds nonstop each arm

TRICEPS
dumbbell kickback
25, 30, and 35 pounds for 10 reps
close grip bench press with barbell
195 pounds for eight, 215 for three sets of six
one-arm dumbbell extension
35, 40, 45 pounds for 10 reps, and 50 pounds for eight
pressdown
three sets of 10 reps with 95 pounds

ABS
pulley knee-ins
45 pounds for four sets of 25 reps
crunches
three sets of 25 reps
hyperextension
two sets of 10 reps

NEGATIVE BODY METAPHOR NIGHTMARE

August 1, 1980, remember looking outside feel sore angry and tired
thinking only eight more weeks of suffering left until Olympia contest
in Australia where I'd win my fourth title, maybe I should have retired
when I thought that, went outside, sat in a lightweight
banana chair right next to the pool, as I sat down the chair and I
slid into the pool, the chair was OK, but I hit my groin on the ledge
smashing my bulbous urethra causing massive bleeding inside
there was blood gushing out of my penis; went rushing to the
hospital where I bled for four hours. Lost over a quart of blood . . .
catheter inserted . . . put on intravenous . . . went into shock . . .
thought I was dying . . . near-death experience felt peaceful . . .
white light all around glowing . . . should I stay or go?
Next thing I know I'm back lying in hospital bed . . .
had good excuse not to compete instead . . . but still did.
Never was more pissed off than this.
Healing, a week later relaxing in bed
looked through Jung's *Memories, Dreams, and Reflections* and read
advice related to my needs; the responsibility for this mishap lay with me
my attitude of not taking mistakes into the big picture a bit crude
no sure road to success, life's always an experiment
and sometimes a complete mess. All I can do
is accept truth in the moment for me.
God only knows what my ultimate fate will be.
In this way I form an ego that is great
capable of dealing with future I don't forsee.

REFRAMING AFTER DISASTER

After okayed by my doctor to begin regaining
what I had lost from this bizarre experience
with only five weeks before Olympia remaining
to put pieces back together in my training
lost 15 pounds bodyweight from accident
now at 190 made decision to compete near that bodyweight
with maximum muscularity . . . why this tragic karmic event?
Could have won if it didn't happen, asked myself
what part did my attitude play in this?
In the hospital remember a dream:

I'm in the house where I spent the first 12 years of my life
at 21 Franklin Street, in the kitchen I hear noise in the living
room and soon find 30 immigrants sitting in a circle in there
I say to them "you are uninvited guests in my home, now get
the hell out of here." As I said this one man stood up and as
I looked at him, he disappeared, then they all left.

What does it all mean?
The accident, the dream, now healing
realizing what brought it all on was me.
Looking back on all of this now
I know the right decision would have been
not to compete in Australia
but listening to my doctor who said it was OK
and to career advice Arnold S. gave me
led to defending my title. Besides, I had my plane ticket anyway.
Now I know why everybody said hindsight is 100 percent.
Think I could have won my fourth Olympia 1981 in Columbus
if I hadn't competed in 1980 but too obsessed with winning
my ego pushed me into defeat
lost touch with inner self
falling from grace
almost bled to death.

WORKOUT 120

Being careful not to start bleeding again, funny now thinking
back, how I was checking my penis every 5 minutes, here's what
I did in my last workouts before leaving for Australia Olympia:
September 24, 1980 did back, biceps, forearms, abs in Palm Springs

barbell row 150, 160, 170 pounds for 10 reps
one-arm dumbbell row three sets of 10 reps with 105 pounds
then top deadlift 255 pounds for 15 reps, 345 for 12, 415 for 10,
checking my penis after every set
and shrugging with dumbbells 95 pounds three sets of 10 reps
and pulldown behind neck 220 pounds for 12, 230 pounds for 10 reps, 240 for eight
then front pulldown 170 for three sets of 8 reps
being careful not to hit myself on the head
that I would hate, after 150, 160, 170 pounds for 10 reps low cable row
was grateful I was not bleeding
then finished lats with three sets of 10 reps with 110 pounds
one-arm cable row and took a short break
because of a headache took 500 mg. of Tylenol

and began working biceps with
dumbbell concentration curl 40 pounds for 10 reps, 45 for 10, 50 for eight drop to 35
pounds for seven
dumbbell 30-degree incline curl 40 pounds for 10 reps, 45 for eight, 45 for seven, drop
to 35 for six
next did drop sets preacher cable curl bench 120 pounds for eight reps, 100 for six, 75
for five,

on to forearms barbell reverse curl 95, 105, 105 pounds for 10 reps
then wrist curl 100 pounds for 15 reps, 90 for 15, 80 for 15, only 20 seconds rest
between sets

Later that night worked abs and lower back
did hyperextension 25 pounds for two sets of 15
then 100 crunches and pulley knee-in 55 pounds for 30 reps, 60 for 25, 65 for 20
penis still not bleeding
then did one-arm cable crunches 120 pounds for 40 reps, 30, 30 and 100 seated twists.

Practiced compulsory poses for 20 or near
30 minutes then went through my free posing routine
three times in the mirror.
That year I learned that just like all men
I am a two-headed being
and made decisions with my big head
while my little head bled
instead should have listened to message my little head said
crying tears of red.

WORKOUT 121

September 25 at 9 A.M. I took photos in backyard; I really looked hard when I viewed them a few days later. Then I got a few hours of sun while on my raft as I floated in the pool. I tanned really dark with no Jantanna dripping down my back to make a mess and no suntanned hands. I began training *thighs* at 4:30 P.M. that day. After which I practiced compulsory posing—holding each pose longer and longer.

one-leg top extension
80 and 90 pounds for 20 reps, 100 for 15 each leg
squat
185, 245, and 285 pounds for 10 reps
lunge
100, 110, and 120 pounds for 10 reps
leg extension
240 pounds for eight reps, 200 and 160 for six with only enough rest between sets to change the weight
leg curl
90 pounds for 10 reps, 95 for nine, 100 for eight, 70 for eight
stiff legged deadlift
two sets of 10 reps with 75 pounds
seated calf raises
100, 110, and 120 pounds for 15 reps
donkeys
(with 230-pound rider), four sets of 15 reps

ABS AND LOWER BACK
hyperextension
two sets of 15 reps with 25 pounds
abdominal crunches
40, 30, and 30 reps
pulley knee-in
60 pounds for 30, 30, 20, and 20 reps
one-arm cable crunch
80 pounds for 40, 30, and 30 reps
seated twist
100 reps
stairclimber
six minutes

1980 PRE-CONTEST DIET

The last weeks before the Olympia on a typical day I ate
a five-egg omelet with three ounces cheese and chicken
two cups of coffee sweetened with aspartame and glycine
eight ounces of chicken and one diet soda
eight tablespoons milk/egg protein powder
another cup of coffee late afternoon with usual sweetening
then for dinner 16 ounces of fish and one lite beer
and megadoses of supplements all day of course:
amino acids in free form, B-complex, C-complex, fat soluble
vitamins A, D, and E, liver extract, digestive enzymes
sterol oils, minerals, and lipotropic agents as well.

WORKOUT 122

My last workout in the U.S. before the 1980 Mr. Olympia contest came on September 27. I got up early, drank coffee. An hour later I ran a 10-minute mile, then rested and ate an omelet, a pound of broiled lean ground beef with another cup of coffee. I trained *chest-delts-triceps* from 10 A.M. to 12:15 P.M.. Afterwards I went through my free posing routine three times and felt I had it all down, thus boosting my confidence.

bench press
145 pounds for 15 reps, 195 for 10, then 235, 240, 245, 250, and 255 for six, all slow negatives

75 degree incline dumbbell press
60 pounds for 10 reps, 65 for nine

60 degree incline dumbbell press
70 pounds for seven reps, 75 for six

45 degree incline dumbbell press
80 pounds for six reps

dumbbell flys (little rest between sets)
60 pounds for three sets of 10 reps

V bar dip
with 20 pounds around my waist, three sets of 15 reps

dumbbell pullover
90 pound for two sets of 12 reps

DELTS

one dumbbell front raise
three sets of 10 reps with 75 pounds

dumbbell side raise
35 pounds three sets of 10 reps

rear cable raise
15 pounds for 12 reps, then 20, 20, 15, and 10 pounds for 10 reps

one-arm side cable raises
20, 25, and 30 pounds for 10 reps, nonstop alternating arms

TRICEPS

dumbbell kickback
30, 35, 40, and 45 pounds for 10 reps

close grip bench press
200 pounds four sets of 10 reps (for outer triceps head)

one-arm dumbbell extension
40 pounds for 10 reps, 45 for eight, 50 for six (for the long rear triceps head)

I checked my penis for bleeding, ate lunch, and got two hours of sun. At 6:30 P.M. I did *lower back-abs* workout:

hyperextension
35 pounds for two sets of 15 reps

hanging leg raises
three sets of 25 reps

crunches
40, 30, and 30 reps

pulley knee-in
60 pounds for 30, 30, 30, and 10 reps

one-arm cable crunch
90 pounds for 40, 30, and 30 reps

seated twist
100 reps

treadmill
10 minutes

TREASURES OF MINE DREAM

After finishing third in Australia had a dream
where I find precious silver statues and jewelry
I've stored deep in a cave long time ago
and forgot they were there
discovering cave with a group of friends
I'm traveling with, anxious to get home
they want some of the treasure
and at first I'm reluctant to give them any saying
"that's a very old precious item that belonged
to my great grandmother"
but later I let them take of the treasure of silver
because there is so much.
I take some too and continue to journey home
and pick out a special silver treasure for Christine
whose presence fills this dream.

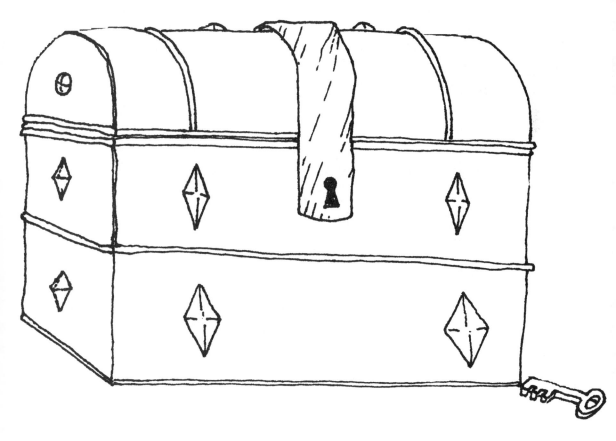

WORKOUT 123

Evenings in Santa Monica in the late 1970s, Christine and I would drive down to Gold's Gym at Third Street. On September 12, in preparation for the 1979 Mr. Olympia contest, we trained *back-biceps-forearms* from 7:45 to past closing at 9:30 P.M.. She was my training partner and did everything I did with lighter weights. That night Christine deadlifted 225 pounds for one rep.

top deadlift
155 pounds for 10 reps, 245 for eight, 295 for six, 315 for five, 315 for five

dumbbell shrug
80, 90, and 100 pounds for 12 reps

one-arm dumbbell row
100 pounds for three sets of 10 reps

barbell row
135, 145, 155, and 165 pounds for 10 reps

front pulldown
190, 200, and 210 pounds for 10 reps

low cable row
140 and 160 pounds for 10 reps

BICEPS
incline dumbbell curl
35 pounds for 10 reps, 40 for 10, 45 for eight, 50 for six

alternate dumbbell curl
50 pounds for seven, 55 for six, 60 for six

one-arm dumbbell concentration curl
40, 45, and 50 pounds for eight reps

FOREARMS (with barbell)
reverse curl
70, 80, and 90 pounds for 10 reps

reverse wrist curl
40, 40,and 50 pounds for 15 reps

wrist curl
85, 115, and 115 pounds for 15 reps

ABS
one-arm cable crunch
two sets of 25 reps with 50 pounds

{**incline knee-ins**
crunches
both three sets of 50 reps

hyperextensions
25 reps

WORKOUT 124

The next evening we trained *legs* in Gold's Gym from 9:15 until 10:29 pm, when all the strange characters had left before closing time so our workout went just fine. A few weeks earlier I had fallen down stairs hurting my hip while filming a TV exercise show, so I couldn't do full squats this night. Afterwards, we drove in our Jeep through the cool ocean air to our home near the beach. We watched TV until about midnight, then retired. In the morning we woke up feeling sore and very tired from this workout.

CALVES
donkeys
with 250 pounds, five sets for 15 to 20 reps
standing calf machine
200, 250, and 300 pounds for 15 reps
calf raises on leg press machine
200, 220, and 240 pounds for 15 reps
one-legged calf raises
four sets of 15 reps with no weight

THIGHS
leg curl
80 and 90 pounds for 10 reps, 100 for eight, 110 for six
barbell lunges
55, 65,and 75 pounds for 10 reps
leg extension
170 and 200 pounds for 10 reps, 220 for eight
quarter squats
225, 245, and 265 pounds for 15 reps

ABS
one-arm cable crunch
90 pounds for 25 reps with each arm
{ **incline knee-in**
three sets of 50 reps
crunches
three sets of 50 reps
hyperextensions
20 reps

WORKOUT 125

Next evening 9 to 11 P.M. we worked *chest-shoulders-triceps* at Gold's again:

bench press
135, 205, and 255 pounds for 10 reps, 280 for seven, 300 for three

incline dumbbell press
80 pounds for 10 reps, 90 for eight, 100 for six, 100 for six

parallel dip
40 pounds for 10 reps, 60 for eight, 80 for six

DELTS

machine press
135 pounds for 10 reps, 145 for eight, 175 for six, 185 for six with slow negatives

one dumbbell front raise
70, 75, and 80 pounds for 10 reps

side dumbbell raises
three sets of 12 reps with 35 pounds

rear delt machine
three sets of 70 pounds for 10 reps

rear delt raise face down on incline bench
four sets of 30 pounds for 10 reps

pec deck
100 pounds for 15 reps, 120 for 12, 140 for 10

dumbbell pullover
95, 110, 110, and 110 pounds for 10 reps

TRICEPS

close grip bench press
135 pounds for 10 reps, 155 for eight, 165 for seven, 175 for six

one-arm dumbbell extension
35, 40, and 45 pounds for eight reps

one-arm cable kickback
three sets of 35 pounds for 10 reps

one-arm side cable raise
15 pounds for two sets of 10 reps

The ab workout was the same as the day before.

TRAINING IN SOLITARY

The next day September 13, 1979
I left for Palm Springs with intention to stay
all the way until the Mr. Olympia competition
in Columbus, Ohio, on October 6th,
realizing that my focus would be best
training in isolation.
When I arrived it was supposed to be a rest day
but I did a little calves, traps, and delts
training for a total of 28 sets anyway.

WORKOUT 126

The following day got sun from 10 to 11:15 A.M. and was in my gym training *back-biceps-forearms* by 1 P.M..

BACK
front chin
three sets of 10 reps
top deadlift
135 pounds for 20 reps, 185 for 18, 225 for 16, 275 for 15, 315 for 12
one-arm dumbbell row
90 pounds for 12 reps, 95 for 11, 100 for 10

BICEPS
incline dumbbell curl
30, 35, 40, and 45 pounds for 10 reps
alternate dumbbell curl
55 pounds for eight reps, 60 for nine, 65 for seven
preacher cable curl
70, 80, and 85 pounds for 10 reps
preacher barbell curl
70 pounds for 10 reps, 75 for nine, 80 for eight
low incline dumbbell curl
three sets of 10 reps with 30 pounds

FOREARMS
barbell wrist curl
80 pounds for 20 reps, 90 for 15, 100 for 15
reverse barbell curl
three sets of 10 reps with 70 pounds

Went outside and got another hour of sun thinking about specific beneficial attributes called "qualities" while floating on my raft in the pool. These are shape, symmetry, aesthetic lines, proportion, muscularity, separation, definition, and size. Was it wise to ignore all these qualities and just to train for size, when quantity is really qualitative?

WORKOUT 127

I remember lying in the sun the same day repeating my affirmation; saying it off and on while keeping my mind under control. It seemed to wander off anyway so my goal was to remember to say this mind formula in idle moments during the day and set up a mental circuit to crowd out negative thinking. After sunbathing, I took a break and twice listened to a motivational audio tape. That evening I was in my gym from 7:30 until 9 P.M. to train *thighs* and *calves.* If I had had my Leg Blaster, my knees and lower back would probably have felt better after this workout:

leg curl
80, 80, 90, and 100 pounds for 10 reps, 100 for eight
lunges
70 and 80 pounds for 10 reps
leg extension
160 pounds for 12 reps, 180 for 11, 200 for 10, 220 for 10, 240 for eight
hack squat
holding 35-pound dumbbells, three sets of 10 reps

CALVES
seated raise
four sets of 20 reps with 100 pounds
standing calf raise
four sets of 20 reps with 250 pounds

ABS
one-arm cable crunch
50 and 60 pounds for 25 reps, and 60 for 15 each arm
hanging knee-ups
four sets of 25 reps
incline knee-in
50 reps
crunches
holding a two-pound dumbbell on my chest for 50 reps
good morning exercise
70 pounds for two sets of 25 reps
stairclimber
four minutes followed by a swim

WORKOUT 128

Last night slept nine hours straight. I awoke the morning of September 15 at 9:30 A.M., took my supplements with a protein drink, sipped a hot cup of coffee, and meditated from 10:10 to 10:30. After sunbathing for two hours, I began *chest* training at 1:15 P.M..

bench press
135, 205, and 255 pounds for 10 reps, 280 for eight, 300 for four
30 degree incline barbell press
135 pounds for 10 reps, 185 for eight, 205 for seven, 215 for six
70 degree incline dumbbell press
60 pounds for 10 reps, 70 for 10, 75 for eight
dips
three sets of 10 reps with a 35-pound plate
standing dumbbell press
drop sets with 50, 45, 40, and 35 pounds for five reps without rest

After a three-minute break:

standing dumbbell press
drop sets with 50 pounds for 6 reps, 45, 40, and 35 pounds for 4 reps
one dumbbell front raise
three sets of 10 reps with 70 pounds
strict dumbbell side raises
20, 25, and 30 pounds for 10 reps
one-arm side cable raises
25, 25, 30, and 35 pounds for 10 reps
two-arm bent over rear delt cable raises
four sets of 12 reps with 20 pounds
rear delt dumbbell raises (face down on steep incline bench)
25 and 30 pounds for 10 reps

Because of a spasm in upper right shoulder blade, lay on ice for 20 minutes and said my mantra 216 times. Then I took a nap and by 9 P.M., I was in the gym again to do more *chest* work plus *triceps*:

decline fly
40 pounds for 12 reps, 45 for 11, 50 for 10
cable crossover
40 pounds for 12 reps, 45 for 11, 50 for 10
dumbbell pullover
80, 90, and 100 pounds for 10 reps to work the anterior serratus
stiff-arm pulldown
80, 90, and 100 pounds for 12 reps

(continued)

TRICEPS

close grip bench press
135 pounds for 10 reps, 185 for eight, 185 for six, 185 for five with slow negatives

overhead cable extension
50 pounds for 12 reps, 60 for 11, 70 for 10

one-arm dumbbell extension drop sets
35 and 30 pounds for five reps, 25 for six with no rest between sets

pressdown
90 pounds for 12 reps, 100 for 10

one-arm side cable raise
25 pounds for 10 reps, 30 for 10

By this time my delts felt so sore all I could do was abs:

hanging knee-ups
40, 30, and 30 reps

crunches
100 reps

one-arm cable crunches
65 and 75 pounds for 25 reps

stairclimber
five minutes

CIRCUITS

A circuit is a three-ring circus
one ring at a time
I say and see in my dreams
asleep in bed and especially
what I say to me all day
goes round and round in my head
most vulnerable time is early A.M.
when first awake what I hear
keeps playing back all day
unresolved dream fragments, radio, TV
I'd rather select my own frequency
singing my own song instead.
A favorite way is to play
my harmonica version of Bach's Brandenburg concerto
Beatles tunes, Aerosmith, Led Zepplin, or blues of John Mayall.
Most of all.

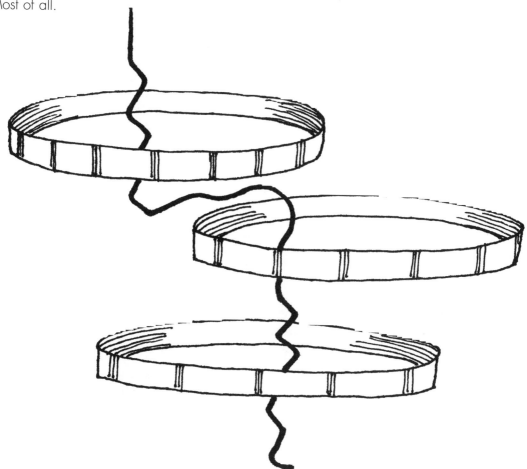

WORKOUT 129

My upper back stiff at 10:40 A.M., so for breakfast I have a protein drink and supplements with an icepack and gram of buffered aspirin. I lie in the sun from 11:45 A.M. to 1 P.M.. For lunch I have turkey, then lie in the sun from 4 to 5 P.M., followed by listening to audiotapes and saying my affirmation while lying on my waterbed. At 8:10 P.M. I begin *back-biceps-forearms* training:

BACK
wide grip front chin
10 reps with no weight, then 10 pounds for 10 reps,
20 for eight, 20 for eight, 25 for seven, 30 for six
barbell row
115, 125, 135, 145, 155, 165, and 175 pounds for 10
reps each set
one-arm dumbbell row
90, 100, and 110 pounds for 10 reps
one-arm lat stretch
one-arm cable row
75 pounds for 12 reps, 85 for 11, 100 for 10
top deadlift
235 pounds for 12, 275 for 10, 315 for eight
dumbbell shrug
80, 90, and 100 pounds for 15 reps
bent over rear delt cable raise
20, 20, and 25 pounds for 10 reps

BICEPS
low incline dumbbell curl
30, 35, 40, and 45 pounds for eight reps, and 50 for
seven
alternate dumbbell curl
55 pounds for eight reps, 60 for seven, 65 for five, 70
for five
barbell preacher curl
60 pounds for 10 reps, 70 for 10, 80 for eight
preacher cable curl
90 pounds for 10 reps, 95 and 100 for eight

FOREARMS (no rest at all between sets)
{
reverse wrist curl
three sets of 10 reps with a 70-pound barbell
barbell wrist curl
three sets of 15 reps with 100 pounds

stairclimber
six minutes

I practiced stomach vacuums for 10 minutes; relaxed and meditated for 20 minutes more; then swallowed aminos, ate a little fruit, and went to bed.

WORKOUT 130

September 17, 1979, from 7:30 to 9:30 P.M. I worked on *calves-thighs-abs*:

CALVES

donkey calf raise
250 pounds for 20 reps, 265 for 18, 275 for 16, 285 for 16, 295 for 16, 300 for 16

one-legged calf raise
three sets of 15 reps holding a 45-pound dumbbell

THIGHS

{ **leg curl**
lunges
both: 80, 90, 100, and 110 pounds for 10 reps

leg extension
180 pounds for 12 reps, 210, 240, and 250 pounds for 10 resting two minutes between sets to do perfect reps

hack squat
three sets of 12 reps with 40-pound dumbbells

ABS

one-arm cable crunch
50, 60, 70, and 80 pounds for 25 reps each arm

incline knee-up
holding 20-pound dumbbell with my feet, four sets of 10 reps

hanging knee-up
strapped a six pound dumbbell between my feet, three sets of 20 reps

KETOGENIC BREAKFAST

Think of the breakfast omelet
tomato avocado cheese
black coffee with artificial sweetening
cottage cheese one scoop
no toast or butter please
used to eat at this ketogenic breakfast
once a week right up until
two weeks before the contest.
Good fats made me stronger
killed hunger and
helped me train heavier and longer.

WORKOUT 131

On September 18, 1979, at 2:10 P.M. I began training *chest-deltoids* for my first workout:

bench press
135, 205, 255, and 280 pounds for 10 reps, 305 pounds for five

30-degree incline press
135 pounds for 10 reps, 185 for 10, 205 for eight

parallel dip
30 pounds for 10 reps, 45 for nine, 60 for eight, 70 for six and slow negatives

DELTS

75 degree incline dumbbell press
60 pounds for 10 reps, 70 for eight, 70 for eight, 70 for nine (I twisted the weights during the press so my palms were facing away from me at the top of the exercise, not locking out my elbows, lowering the weights so that my slowly twisting palms were now facing me at bottom of the press.)

one-arm side cable raise
30, 35, and 40 pounds for 10 reps each arm

one-arm dumbbell side raise
20, 25, and 25 pounds for 10 reps

rear cable raise
pyramiding, or working up in weight each set, then going down in weight: 20, 25, 25, 25, 20, 20, 20, and 20 pounds for 10 reps

My second workout that day began at 8 P.M.:

{ **decline fly**
40, 50, and 60 pounds for 10 reps

cable crossover
40, 45, and 50 pounds for 10 reps

TRICEPS

close grip bench press
135 pounds for 10 reps, 185 for five slow reps, 205 for four with even slower reps

dumbbell pullover
three sets of 90 pounds for 10 reps

one-arm dumbbell extension
35, 40, 45, 50, and 55 pounds for 10 reps

one-arm cable kickback
20, 25, 30, and 35 pounds for 10 reps each arm

ABS

one-arm cable crunch
70 and 75 pounds for 25 reps each arm

{ **incline knee-in**
crunches
both two sets of 50 reps

hyperextension
20 pounds for 20 reps

It was 9:30 P.M. so I quit, went to the high school track and ran a mile in 9 minutes. Feeling really tired by 11 P.M., I went to bed.

SONG OF AFFIRMATION

That night woke up at 4 A.M.
and wrote lyrics to a song:
Ah me the butterfly
gliding above the sun
Ah me da ha bia
means yes oh golden one
Ah me da ko ta
my friend and ally
also called the Sioux
Ah me da boot soo
praise good in you
Ah me that I gotta do too.

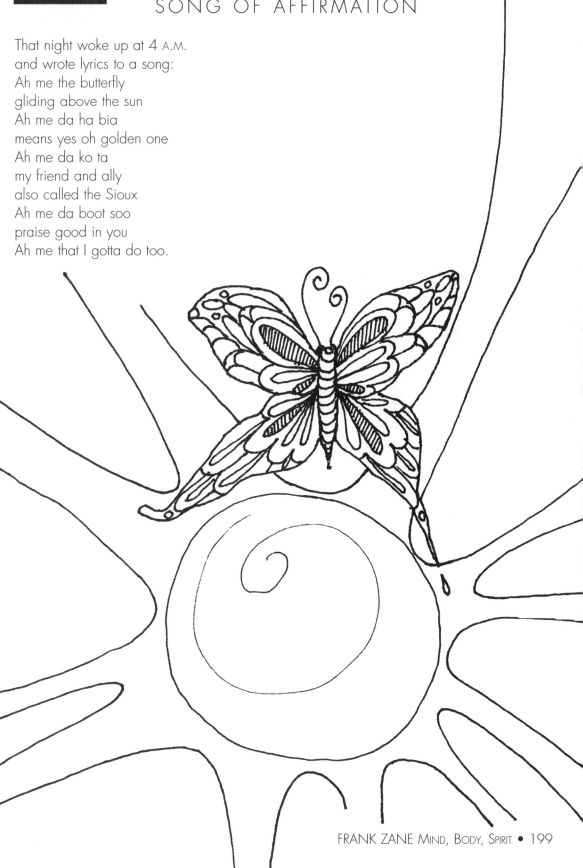

WORKOUT 1 3 2

On September 19, 1979, between 3 and 4:30 P.M. I trained *back-biceps-forearms*. Christine deadlifted 235 pounds easily proving how strong she was to me.

BACK
front chins
no weight for 10 reps, 10 pounds for 10 reps, 20 for nine, 20 for eight, 30 for eight, 30 for seven
bent over barbell row
115, 125, 135, 145, 155, and 165 pounds for 10 reps, 175 for eight
one-arm dumbbell row
100, 110, and 120 pounds for 10 reps
one-arm cable row
75 pounds for 12 reps, 85 for 12, 95 for 10
one-arm lat stretch
dumbbell shrugs
90 pounds for 15 reps, 100 for 12, 110 for 12
bent over rear delt cable raise
three sets of 10 reps with 20 pounds
donkey calf raises
250 pounds for 25 reps, 275 for 22, 285 for 23

BICEPS
incline dumbbell curl
30 pounds for 10 reps, 35 for 10, 40 for 10, 45 for eight, 50 for six
alternate dumbbell curl
55 pounds for 10 reps, 60 for eight, 65 for seven

Feeling pain in my left front delt, I applied a little dmso. Its warm sensation helped me continue.

preacher cable curl
90, 100, and 100 pounds for eight reps

FOREARMS
reverse barbell curl
75, 80, 85,and 90 pounds for 10 reps
barbell wrist curl
90, 100, 110, and 120 pounds for 20 reps
reverse wrist curl
three sets of 15 reps with 30, 40, 40 pounds

ABS
one-arm cable crunch
80 and 85 pounds for 25 reps
{ **incline knee-ins**
crunches
both: two sets of 50 reps
good morning exercise
40 pounds for 20 reps

WORKOUT 133

September 21, 1979, I worked *calves-thighs-abs*.

donkeys
  275 pounds for 24 reps, 300 for 13, iced a cramp
  before continuing with 300 for 15, 300 for 20, 300 for
  20, 300 for 18, 300 for 16, 300 for 14
leg curl
  90 pounds for 10 reps, 100 for nine, 100 for nine, 100
  for 10
lunges
  70, 80, 90, 100 pounds for 10 reps
leg extension
  210 pounds for 12 reps, then 240 and 250 for 10
hack squat
  three sets of 10 reps with 50 pound dumbbells
one-legged top extension
  nine reps with 90 pounds

  ABS
one-arm cable crunch
  90, 90, 100, and 100 pounds for 25 reps each arm
{ **incline knee-in**
crunches
  both two sets of 50 reps
stairclimber
  two minutes for two sets

I got about two hours sun, applied ice to my shoulder two or three times, listened to alpha wave beat frequency audio tape. Later I bought a large light blue roll of paper and installed it in my living room for a photographic background, to take progress photos with Christine.

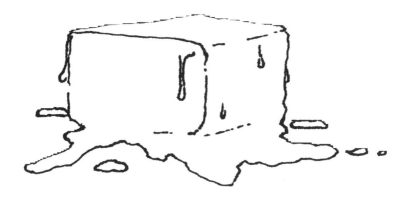

WORKOUT 134

On September 24, 1979, I worked *chest-delts-triceps* from 9:30 A.M. to noon. I said my mantra for a half-hour right before workout, then continued it all the way through:

bench press
135, 185, 225, and 255 pounds for 10 reps, and 275 for 6

incline barbell press
135, 175, and 195 pounds for 10 reps, 210 pounds for seven

dip
10 reps with 20 pounds around my waist, then 30 pounds for 10, 40 for 10, 50 for eight

decline dumbbell fly
40, 45, and 50 pounds for 10 reps

cable crossover
40, 50, and 60 pounds for 10 reps

dumbbell pullover
85, 100, and 100 pounds for 10 reps

pressdown
75 pounds for ten reps, 85 for eight, 90 for seven

DELTS

70 degree incline dumbbell press
50 pounds for 10 reps, 60 for 10, 70 for eight, 75 for seven

one-arm side cable raises
25, 30, and 35 pounds for 10 reps each arm (right front delt began to hurt again)

dumbbell side raises
20, 25, and 30 pounds for 10 reps made me forget the pain

bent over rear delt cable raises
15, 20, 20, 20, 20, and 20 pounds for 10 reps

TRICEPS

close grip bench press
135 pounds for 10 reps, 175 for nine, 195 for eight

one-arm dumbbell extension
30 pounds for 10 reps, 35 for 10, 40 for nine

one-arm cable kickback
35, 40, and 50 pounds for 10 reps

EZ bar seated triceps extension
60, 70, and 80 pounds for 10 reps

After a break, I resumed the workout at 7 P.M.:

one-leg top extension
60 pounds for 16 reps, 70 for 15, 80 for 12, 90 for 10

lunges
70, 80, and 90 pounds for 10 reps

ABS

one-arm cable crunch
two sets of 50 reps with 75 pounds for each arm

{ **incline knee-in**
crunches
both: three sets of 50 reps

I ended the workout practicing stomach vacuums interspersed with one-arm lat stretch.

REST TODAY AFTER YESTERDAY

At the end of the day
evaluated my stay in the gym.
Wrote down entire workout from memory
quote "It was a good session, strong in everything
but didn't push heavier because left front deltoid hurt
from under arm to top of shoulder joint."
Writing this made
my delts feel pumped and bigger.
Rested today,
got adjustment at chiropractor
ultrasound made delt feel better.

WORKOUT 135

September 26, 1979, I did a *back-biceps-forearms* workout from 9 to 11 A.M.:

BACK
one-arm dumbbell row
70, 85, 100, 110, and 120 pounds for 10 reps
one-arm lat stretch
one-arm cable row
110, 110, and 125 pounds for 10 reps
barbell row
135 pounds for 12 reps, 155 for 12, 165 for 10, 175 for 10, 185 for 10
top deadlift
205 and 255 pounds for 10 reps, 305 for six but twisted L-5 lumbar vertebra so stopped and iced
dumbbell shrug
three sets of 10 reps with 90-pound dumbbells
rear delt cable raise
15 pounds three sets of 15 reps

BICEPS
preacher curl
60 pounds for eight, 70 for nine, 75, 80, and 85 for eight
low incline curl
30 pounds for 10 reps, 35 for 10, 40 for eight
preacher cable curl
80, 90, 100, and 110 pounds for 10 reps

FOREARMS
reverse wrist curl
50 pounds for three sets of 15 reps
wrist curl
100 pounds for three sets of 15 reps

ABS (from 9 to 10 P.M.)
pulley knee-in
15, 20, 25, and 30 pounds for 25 reps, rested, then did it again
crunch
four sets of 50 reps
one-arm cable crunch
two sets of 25 reps with 75 pounds
seated twists
100 reps
hyperextensions
20, 15, and 10 reps

That night Christine deadlifted 135 pounds for eight reps, 155 for five, 175 for three, 195 for two, then one rep each at 205, 215, 225, 240, 245, and 250 pounds without letting me tell her the weight before she did it.

WORKOUT 136

After spending most of September 27, 1979, sunbathing, I trained *legs* from 8:30 to 10 P.M..

CALVES
donkeys
250 pounds for 30 reps, 275 for 25, 300 for 20, 325 for 16, 335 for 15

THIGHS
leg curl
90, 100, 100, and 100 pounds for 10 reps
lunges
70, 80, 90, and 100 pounds for 10 reps
leg extension
210 pounds for 12 reps, 240 for 10, 265 for eight, without rest drop to 180 pounds for eight reps

ABS
pulley knee-in
35 pounds five sets of 25 reps
crunches
three sets of 50 reps
one-arm cable crunches
two sets of 50 reps
seated twist
100 reps

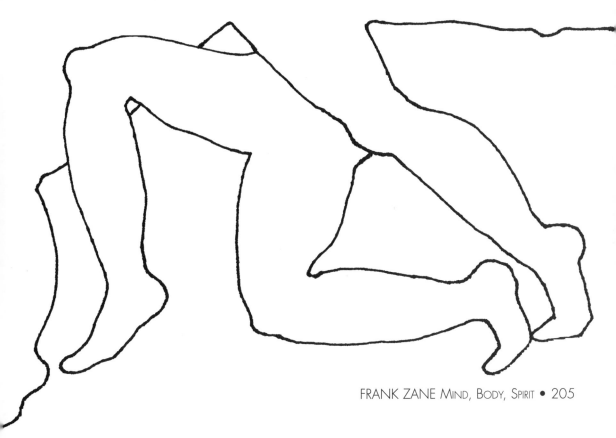

WORKOUT 137

On September 28, 1979, from 10 A.M. to 12:30 P.M. I did *chest-delts-triceps-abs*:

CHEST
bench press
135 pounds for 12 reps, 185 for 10, 225 for 10, 275 for six
low incline barbell press
135 pounds for 10 reps, 185 for 10, 205 for eight, 215 for six
dips
20, 40, and 60 pounds for 10 reps, 70 for eight
front chin with wide grip
five sets of 10 reps
decline fly
40, 50, and 55 pounds for 10 reps
cable crossover
65, 70, and 60 pounds for 10 reps
pullover
100 pounds three sets of 10 reps

DELTS
70 degree incline bench
60 pounds for 10 reps, 70 for eight, 70 for eight
one dumbbell front raise
60 pounds for 12 reps, 65 for 12, 70 for 10, 75 for eight
side cable raise
15 pounds for 12 reps, 20 for 12, 25 for 10, 30 for 10
rear delt cable raise
15, 20, and 25 pounds for 10 reps
dumbbell shrug
80, 90, and 95 pounds for 20 reps

TRICEPS
close grip bench press
155 pounds for 10 reps, 185 for 10, 205 for four slow reps
one-arm dumbbell extension
30 pounds for 10 reps, 35 for nine, 40 for eight, 45 for eight
one-arm cable kickback
45 pounds for three sets of 10 reps
seated EZ bar extension
70 pounds for three sets of 10 reps

My delts were really sore after all of this, so iced them out for over one hour. Later I bought Christine flowers and a golden Buddha. I returned to the gym at 10 P.M..

ABS
pulley knee-in
40 pounds for five sets of 25 reps
crunches
three sets of 50 reps
seated twists
100 reps
stationary bike
20 minutes

SUMMER WORKOUTS IN RETROSPECT

DATE	MY WORKOUT	YOUR WORKOUT
June 22	back, biceps, forearms, abs	
June 24	thighs, calves, abs	
June 26	delts, chest, triceps, abs	
June 28	back, biceps, forearms, abs	
June 30	thighs, calves, abs	
July 2	delts, chest, triceps, abs	
July 4	back, biceps, forearms, abs	
July 5	thighs, calves	
July 7	chest, shoulders, triceps, abs	
July 10	chest, back, triceps	
July 11	thighs, calves, abs	
July 13	delts, biceps, forearms, aerobics	
July 15	back, chest, triceps, abs	
July 16	thighs, calves, abs	
July 18	delts, biceps, forearm, aerobics, abs	
July 20	chest, back, triceps, delts, abs	
July 22	back, biceps, forearms	
July 23	thighs, calves, abs	
July 24	chest, triceps, delts, abs, aerobics	
July 26	back, biceps, forearms	
July 27	calves, thighs, abs	
July 28	chest, shoulders, triceps, abs	
July 30	back, biceps, forearms, abs	
July 31	thighs, calves, abs, aerobics	
August 2	chest, triceps, delts, abs, aerobics	
August 4	back, biceps, forearms, abs	
August 5	aerobics, calves, thighs, abs	
August 7	chest, triceps, delts, abs	
August 9	aerobics, back, biceps, forearms, abs	

August 10	calves, thighs, abs, aerobics
August 11	chest, shoulders, triceps, abs
August 13	back, biceps, forearms, abs
August 14	aerobics, thighs, calves, abs
August 16	chest, shoulders, triceps, abs
August 18	back, biceps, forearms, abs, aerobics
August 19	calves, thighs, abs
August 20	chest, shoulders, triceps, abs, aerobics
August 22	back, biceps, forearms, abs
August 23	thighs, calves, abs, aerobics
August 24	chest, shoulders, triceps, abs
August 27	back, biceps, forearms, abs
August 28	thighs, calves, abs
August 30	chest, shoulders, triceps abs
September 1	back, biceps, forearms, abs
September 2	calves, thighs, abs
September 3	chest, shoulders, triceps, abs
September 5	back, biceps, forearms, abs
September 6	thighs, calves, abs
September 7	chest, shoulders, triceps, abs, aerobics
September 9	back, biceps, forearms, aerobics, abs
September 10	calves, thighs, abs
September 12	chest, delts, triceps, abs, aerobics
September 14	back, biceps, forearms, abs
September 15	calves, thighs, abs, aerobics
September 16	chest, delts, triceps, abs
September 18	back, biceps, forearms, abs
September 19	thighs, calves, abs
September 20	chest, shoulders, triceps, abs

MY HOUSE

Building the body
my house the archetype
foundation, floors, walls,
fireplace, chimney, windows, halls
this house is my body built by repitition.
Building I learn new skills
time labor saving secrets
forget all the frills
I want a basic place to live
that way there's less to wear away
year after year.
Material possessions keeps adding stuff
if my house is never finished
its because I still don't have enough.
Yet as I move from floor to floor
sense the energy feeling I am my building
and what I need is less, not more.

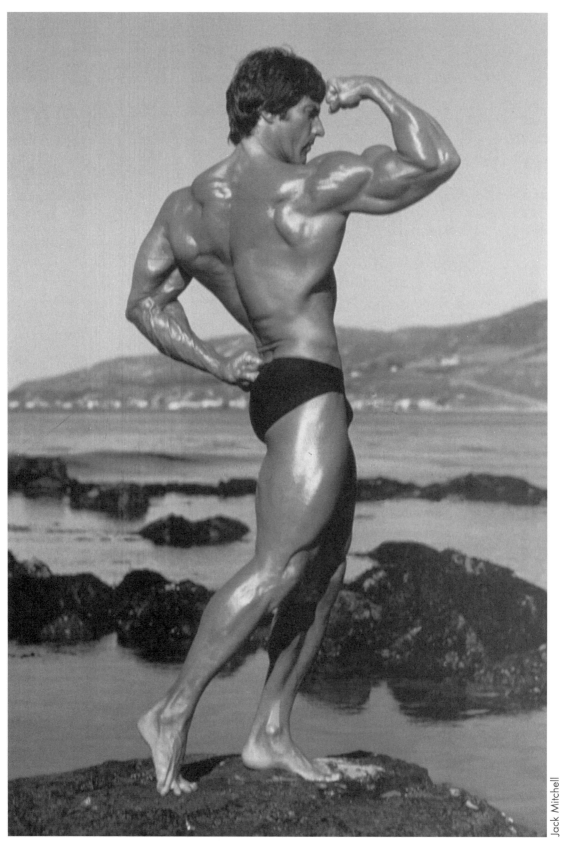

AUTUMN DIARY

I live and work in the house of me
though each room is different I'm the same
kitchen, gym, bedroom, walkways
eat, train, sleep here make gains
visitors welcomed don't complain
me and you share the same house too.

WHAT IS FAITH?

Faith is expressed in different degrees
most think it's belief in things unseen
what hasn't happened yet
with right attitude maybe will transpire
how we hope
but
beyond this blind belief exists
highest level of faith
means being sure
100 percent certain
confident expectation
in the know
living it before it occurs
as above so below
answers found in prayer
tell us so.
This example of faith comes to mind
where in the Bible I find
Matthew 8: 5-13
this army captain comes up to Christ
says his servant is lying ill in paralysis
Christ replies "I will come and heal him."
Captain answers "Sir, I am not fit
to have you under my roof only say the word
and my servant will be cured."
When Jesus heard this he marveled
and said to his followers
"I tell you truly never have I met
faith like this anywhere in Israel."
Then he replied to the Captain
"Go you have faith your prayer is answered."
In western culture
we take something on faith
until we know for certain
but what really exists
behind the uncertain
curtain will show
in highest faith
what we already know.

WORKOUT 138

With competition day one week away, my last three workouts Sunday, Monday, and Tuesday needed to be my very best. I practiced compulsory posing for one hour; holding each pose 45 seconds without shaking. Then I got in an hour of sunbathing—standing with my eyes closed while facing the sun and imagining I was already on stage, thighs and abs tensed always. All day I silently repeated my mantra. From 7 to 9 P.M. I worked on *back-biceps-forearms-abs*. That evening Christine did her best deadlift so far: 155 pounds for five reps, 185 for two, then 215, 235, 255 pounds for one rep.

BACK
bent over rowing
115, 135, 155 pounds for 12 reps, 175 for 10, 185 for eight
front chin
no weight for 10 reps, then 10, 20, and 25 pounds for 10 reps
rear delt cable raise
15, 20, 25, and 15 pounds for 10 reps, rest 1 minute, then 25 and 15 pounds for 10 reps
one-arm dumbbell row
100, 120, and 120 pounds for 10 reps
one-arm cable row
110, 125, and 135 pounds for 10 reps

BICEPS
barbell preacher curl
55 and 65 pounds for 10 reps, 70, 70, and 70 pounds for eight reps
incline dumbbell curl
30 pounds for 10 reps, 35 for nine, 35 for nine
one-arm seated dumbbell curl
nonstop each arm: 50 pounds for 10 reps, 45 for 10, 40 for nine, 35 for eight

FOREARMS
reverse curl
60, 70, and 80 pounds for 10 reps
wrist curl
80, 90, and 100 pounds for 15 reps both with barbell

ABS
pulley knee-in
40 pounds around my feet did four sets of 25 reps
crunches
40, 30, and 30 reps
seated twist
100 reps
stairclimber
three minutes

WORKOUT 139

I took 40 amino acid and 80 liver extract capsules with small bits of food throughout the day. This low caloric super-energy jolt fueled my training as my mantra crowded out negative thinking. From 8:45 to 10:05 P.M. I did the following *calves-abs* workout in the gym.

CALVES

donkeys
250 pounds for 30 reps, 360 for 15, 250 for 10, rest 1 minute, then 360 for 15, 250 for 10, rest one minute again, then 360 for 15, 250 for nine, rest, 360 for 16, 250 for nine

leg curl
100 and 110 pounds for eight reps, 120 for seven

lunges
100, 120, 130 pounds for 10 reps

leg extension
210 and 240 pounds for 10 reps, 265 for nine. This was the heaviest I ever did

ABS

pulley knee-in
40 pounds for five sets of 25 reps

crunches
three sets of 50 reps

one-arm cable crunch
75 pounds each arm two sets of 25 reps

hyperextension
25 reps

seated twist
100 reps

WORKOUT 140

Before training I got in a few hours of sun. My golden copper-hued skin glistened in the photographs taken late in the afternoon. Eating at the House of Lamb three hours before the workout made my training easier. Afterwards I posed intensely visualizing my stage presentation and realizing that I'd accomplished my goal: over-trained four days before I competed on stage. All I had to do now was rest, stay confident, sun, practice posing in order to look my all time best . . . and I did. From 7:30 to 10:20 P.M. this last *chest-shoulder-triceps* workout before contest was fast-paced with little rest between sets, cultivating a breathless state.

CHEST

bench press
135 pounds for 12 reps, 185 for 10, 235 for 10, 265 for eight

low incline barbell press
135, 185, and 205 pounds for 10 reps

dips
20 pounds for 10 reps, 50 for 10, 70 for eight

decline fly
45, 55,and 65 pounds for 10 reps

cable crossover
75, 60, and 60 pounds for 10 reps

DELTS

dumbbell press
60 pounds for nine, 70 for eight, 70 for eight

one-dumbbell front raise
60, 70, and 75 pounds for 10 reps

one-arm side cable raise
15, 20, and 25 pounds for 10 reps

rear delt cable raise
15, 20, and 20 pounds for 10 reps, 15 pounds for 12 reps

wide grip chin
zero pounds for 12 reps, 10 for 12, 20 for 10, 25 for 10

dumbbell shrug
three sets of 20 reps with 100 pounds

one-arm cable row
125, 135, and 145 pounds for 10 reps to add lower lat finishing touches and maximize serratus for stomach vacuum pose

dumbbell pullover
three sets of 100 pounds for 10 reps

stiff-arm pressdown using lat machine
three sets of 75 pounds for 10 reps

TRICEPS

one-arm dumbbell extension
30 pounds for 10 reps, 35 for 10, 40 for eight, 45 for six

one-arm cable kickback
50 pounds for 10, eight, and six reps

EZ bar overhead extensions
three sets of eight reps with 70 pounds

(continued)

BICEPS

one-arm dumbbell concentration curl
30, 35, and 40 pounds for 10 reps

ABS

pulley knee-in
50 pounds for 25, 25, 15, 10, 10, eight, and seven reps
crunches
four sets of 25 reps
seated twist
100 reps
stairclimber
three minutes

MY POSING ROUTINE

October 3, 1979 Wednesday
got two hours morning sun
then drove to L.A.
repeating my mantra all the way
I have already won
focused on bliss in the time remaining
packed feeling tired, got an adjustment
from Dr. Hexberg, my chiropractor
relaxed, practiced my posing routine
I called them by special names:

1. front right overhead fists
2. back 3/4 double biceps
3. front left biceps right hip
4. left hip most muscular
5. back 3/4 reaching for it
6. front left behind neck right biceps
7. left side triceps
8. back left biceps right overhead
9. back left biceps right behind neck fingers spread
10. left fist right hip most muscular
11. lunging front double biceps
12. lunging front left behind neck right biceps
13. lunging front left biceps right overhead
14. kneeling back 3/4 lat spread
15. left front overhead with vacuum
16. right most muscular hands on hips
17. right front overhead fingers extended abs
18. left front biceps right overhead abs
19. left front abs hands behind head
20. vacuum hands behind head

Twenty poses in all not too long
not too short
on and off the stage in three minutes flat
hold each pose five to seven seconds without shaking
energy builds each pose more forceful
out of the air hands snatch victory
all muscles tense but with relaxed face
no visible signs of heavy breathing
enjoying it really looks easy.
In my mind could hear the crowd screaming.

MORE POSING

Caught plane for Columbus TWA from LA
with Christine at 10:35 A.M.
leaned back relaxed thought
about Arnold's contest saying
"When I get on the plane I'm already on vacation"
simultaneously while mantra kept repeating
purifying my perception arriving at airport
driving in a white limousine
passed Holiday Inn billboard reading
"Welcome Frank Zane Mr. Olympia."
Everybody else saw it too on their way into town.
Later relaxing in hotel room thought
how posing is a show of pride, even arrogance
rhythmic muscular bare elegance condensed
a list of novel movements in a sequence
resolving Narcissus complex
once and for all
not for mirror but for audience
muscles tensed
relaxed face
feeling ease
crowd pleasing confidence
faith in winning a show of strength
supposing posture attitude transposing
wide structure all encompassing
full range of human emotion
there's front double biceps: balance
lat spread front and rear
breath and force don't dare come near
aerodynamic wings fly away with wind
most muscular crab compact scary in fact
striations vascularity details intact
I see in overhead shots, victory
expanding soul free life's mystery
side chest pose swelling with pride
why hide it pigeons won't
side triceps best wily profile
don't forget jutting leg biceps
and abdominal pose
ridges arose
in a rock garden of symmetry
majesty twisting back 3/4 hardest back double biceps pose
from the side always a small waist
in everybody's face.

LAST DAY BEFORE COMPETITION

By Friday still had eaten little carbs
so for 8 A.M. breakfast had four poached eggs and a steak
with supplements and a psyllium drink
my intestinal lubricant
for noon lunch had 12 ounces fish and steamed vegetables
in a restaurant in German section of Columbus
for dinner two chicken breasts eight ounces of fish and a salad
three hours later ate a filet steak and half a small baked yam.
Still practicing posing looking more and more defined, said to myself
all I can do now is relax
feel at ease knowing I'd won
starting giving thanks ahead of time
made a mental list of appreciation
after all I was in shape through sacrifice
not only mine
but mostly my wife's
putting her life on hold
so I could win.

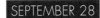

THE BIG DAY

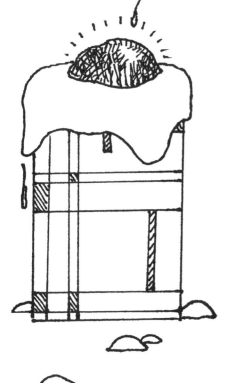

Saturday October 6, 1979, awoke, ate breakfast
at 8 A.M. had one piece calves liver, three poached eggs
coffee and a small baked yam
relaxed on my bed blindfolded resting my eyes
visualizing success instead
and every 45 minutes had
three ounces baked yam
and amino acids right up to noon
then a little expresso
and left for the show
prejudging one to four P.M.
then rested, ate steak and a baked potato
at a restaurant, relaxed until 7 P.M.
went back to the show feeling best ever
knew I'd win when everyone was on stage together
postures of excellence won Mr. Olympia number three.
After the show at the banquet
Mike Mentzer told me
"It wasn't your fault that you won."
I appreciated the gesture
after all was said and done.

REFLECTION THE WEEK AFTER WINNING

Contemplating what I did to win
here's what I wrote in my diary then:
What I developed along with my body
was a kind of consciousness or awareness
developed through weight training, meditation
and paying attention to dreams where
I learned to pick and resonate with
vibrations in my environment.
No difference between me and this
environment because I'm in resonance
with it, a part of it, not different from
and not only do
I create my own environment
but the environment creates me, too
since there is no fundamental difference
between me and it.
So self power is an illusion.
All that exists is other power
and I open myself to the universe.
Discriminating a separate self
is nothing more than splitting off
chunks of other power.

SEPTEMBER 30

HARVEST GLORY

Insight is preceded by preparation
just as in autumn
the harvest is ready
after months of laborious summer
insight ripens and suddenly blooms
in a dream or in waking
like winning Mr. Olympia
my dream come true.
Now my training trend
had come to completion

I've peaked by going through
all seasons of training
winter maintenance
growth in spring
intensity of summer
the colors of autumn leaves
are brightest just before they fall.
Can't help thinking about
"time to fall is time to float for a lotus
    blossom."

WORKOUT 141

One week without training is the longest break I can take to stay in shape, so why give it up after all that work anyway? I went back to my regular workouts using just enough weight to get a good pump. Late one evening at Gold's Gym I did this workout for *back-biceps-forearms*:

BACK
top deadlift
  185 pounds for 10 reps, 225 for 10, 275 for eight, 325 for six
dumbbell shrug
  three sets with 100 pounds for 10 reps
barbell bent over row
  135, 155, and 175 pounds for 10 reps
low cable row
  150, 170, and 190 pounds for 10 reps
pulldown behind neck
  190 and 200 pounds for 10 reps
rear delt machine
  two sets of 12 reps with 60 pounds

BICEPS
dumbbell concentration curl
  30, 40, and 45 pounds for 10 reps
preacher curl
  60- 65- and 70-pound barbell for 10 reps
face down incline dumbbell curl
  three sets of 10 reps with 30 pounders

FOREARMS
barbell wrist curl
  three sets with 100 pounds for 12 reps
barbell reverse curl
  two sets with 70 pounds for 10 reps

ABS
{ **incline knee-in**
crunches
  both: two sets of 50 reps
hyperextensions
  20 reps

WORKOUT 142

The following day I did a *leg* workout at Gold's from 9:30 to 10:30 P.M.. The next morning I weighed 198 pounds.

THIGHS
leg extension
160 pounds for 12 reps, 180 for 10, 200 for nine
lunges
60, 70, and 80 pounds for 10 reps
leg curl
80 pounds for 10 reps, 90 for 10, 100 for eight
donkey calf raise (with a 220-pound rider)
five sets of 20 reps

ABS
{ **knee-ins**
crunches
both two sets of 50 reps
hyperextensions
20 reps

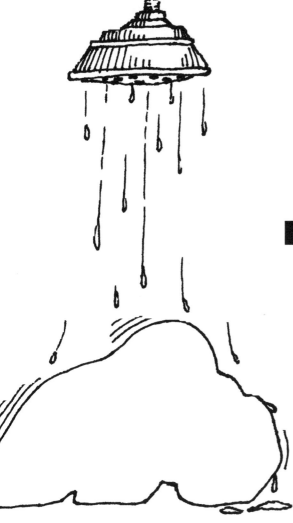

OCTOBER 3

MIGHT AS WELL TRAIN ANYWAY

Over the years I've come to the conclusion
my body is sore whether I train or not.
This is no mere illusion
no matter what time of the year, cold or hot
might as well train anyway
and since I need to shower everyday
at least with weight training
I'll build my body this way
and pain can be voluntary.

FRANK ZANE MIND, BODY, SPIRIT • 223

WORKOUT 143

My next workout came two days later in Palm Springs after relaxing and sunning in this cooler October weather. For 7 to 8 P.M. I hit *chest-shoulders-triceps*. A few days later Christine did her best deadlifting, a 350-pound top deadlift from knees up on power rack and two reps with 270 pulled up from the floor—surely with one rep she could have even done more.

low incline bench press
  135, 185, and 205 pounds for 10 reps
dips
  slow negative weighted 20 pounds for eight reps, 30 for seven, 40 for six
cable crossover
  60 pounds for 10 reps, 70 for 10, 80 for nine

  DELTS
dumbbell press
  50 pounds for 12 reps, 60 for 10
one-arm side cable raise
  15, 20, and 25 pounds for 10 reps each arm, no rest between sets
bent over rear delt cable raise
  15 pounds for 12 reps, 20 for 11, 25 for 10, 15 for 10
dumbbell pullover
  two sets of 12 reps with 85 pounds
one-arm dumbbell extension
  30 pounds for 10 reps, 35 for 10, 40 for eight
EZ bar seated overhead extension
  two sets of 10 reps with 80 pounds
one-arm cable kickback
  30, 30, and 25 pounds for 10 reps nonstop each arm

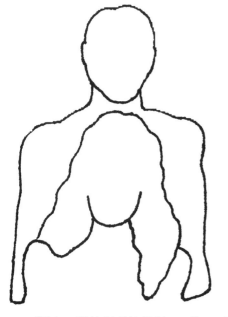

THE ANIMA ARCHETYPE

Today I read about the archetypes
Anima and Animus by Carl Jung's wife
Emma says the woman in man
is called anima, his image of the feminine
new undertakings new discoveries
are brought to man's consciousness by this divine being
living inside his collective unconsciousness
anima sings an emotional stirring
call it intuition, it's what women are about
in my dreams my heart soul with wings
this anima shouts to me
new possibilities.

WORKOUT 144

Feeling great, I begin a *back-biceps-forearm* workout at 8 P.M. starting with:

BACK
front pulldown
160, 180, and 200 pounds for 10 reps
low cable row
160, 170, and 180 pounds for 10 reps
one-arm dumbbell row
80, 85, 90 pounds for 10 reps
close grip pulldown
130, 150, and 160 pounds for 10 reps

BICEPS
alternate dumbbell curl
35, 40, 45 pounds for 10 reps
preacher cable curl
100 pounds for 12 reps, 110 for 11, 125 for seven
low incline curl
30 pounds for 10 reps, 35 for seven, 40 for seven

FOREARMS
barbell reverse curl
70 and 70 pounds for 10 reps
wrist curl
90 and 90 pounds for 15 reps

ABS
incline leg raise
crunches
both: four sets of 25 reps
treadmill
12 minutes

WORKOUT 145

The next day I rode my bike for 30 minutes in the cool morning dawn of late October. Then after relaxing a bit, I ate three soft boiled eggs on two pieces toast with coffee. An hour later I went into my gym for a *leg* workout.

leg extension
   160 pounds for 15, 180 pounds for 12, 200 pounds for 10

lunge
   70, 80, and 90 pounds for 12

leg curl
   80, 90, and 100 pounds for 10

   CALVES
one-legged raise
   holding 20- 30- and 40-pound dumbbell for 15

seated calf raise
   three sets of 15 reps with 100 pounds

donkey calf raise
   three sets of 15 reps with 240 pounds

   ABS
{ **incline leg raise**
   crunches
   both three sets of 30 reps

seated twists
   100 nonstop reps

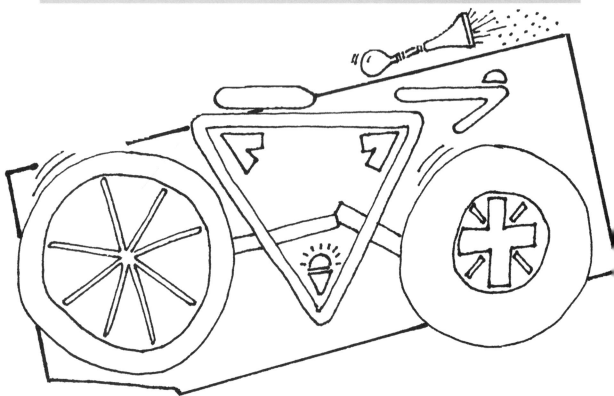

WORKOUT 146

Next day from 9 to 11 A.M. I worked *chest-shoulders-triceps* with a powerlifting friend who had bench pressed 620 pounds. His presence pushed my poundages:

CHEST
bench press
140 pounds for 12 reps, 190 for nine, 230 for five, 250 for two, 270 for one, with real slow negatives
low incline press
140 pounds for 10 reps, 180 for six, 200 for three, with slow negatives
dumbbell press
60 pounds for 10 reps, 65 for eight, 70 for six
dumbbell fly
45 pounds for 10 reps, 55 for nine, 60 for eight
dumbbell pullover (lying across flat bench)
75, 80, and 85 pounds for 10 reps

TRICEPS
dumbbell kickbacks
25 pounds for 15 reps, 30 for 12, 35 for 10
one-arm dumbbell extension
35 pounds for 10 reps, 40 for nine, 45 for seven
pressdown
80 pounds for 15 reps, 100 for 12, 110 for 10

DELTS
bent over rear delt cable raise
10 pounds for 15 reps, 15 for 12, 15 for 12
one-arm side cable raises
15 pounds for 12 reps, 20 for 11, 20 for 10, nonstop each arm

ABS
pulley knee-in
with weight around my ankles of 35 pounds for 30 reps, 40 for 25, 45 for 25, 50 for 20
crunches
three sets of 30 reps
hyperextensions
20 reps
seated twists
100 reps

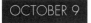

OCTOBER

October is the glory of autumn
nature's expressly designed statement
like this body's planned consequence
defines this month's events
with a wonderful story

leaves orange red and yellow
this communal hymn
begins to fall
around my home
and my gym.

WORKOUT 147

Back in the summer 1969 I did one of my first workouts with Arnold, the best training partner around. We trained *chest-back*.

WARM-UP
cleans and overhead presses
two sets of 15 reps on 70 and 80 pounds

CHEST
bench press
135, 185, 225, 255, and 275 pounds for eight to 10 reps
front chin
five sets of 10 reps
35-degree incline barbell press
135, 185, and 225 pounds for eight to 10 reps

dumbbell fly
three sets of 10 reps with 60 pounds
dumbbell pullover across the bench
90, 100, 105, and 110 pounds for 10 reps
cable crossover
three sets of 12 reps, with little rest between sets, all the time doing doorway stretch
T-bar row
three 45-pound plates on the end of the Olympic bar for three sets of 10 reps (Arnold used four, five, and six plates)
low cable row
170, 180, and 190 pounds for 10 reps
one-arm dumbbell row
90, 95, and 100 pounds for 10 reps
behind neck pulldown
three sets of 10 reps with 180, 190, 200 pounds

ABS
crunches
100 reps
seated twists
100 reps
flat leg raise
two sets of 50 reps

MR. WORLD

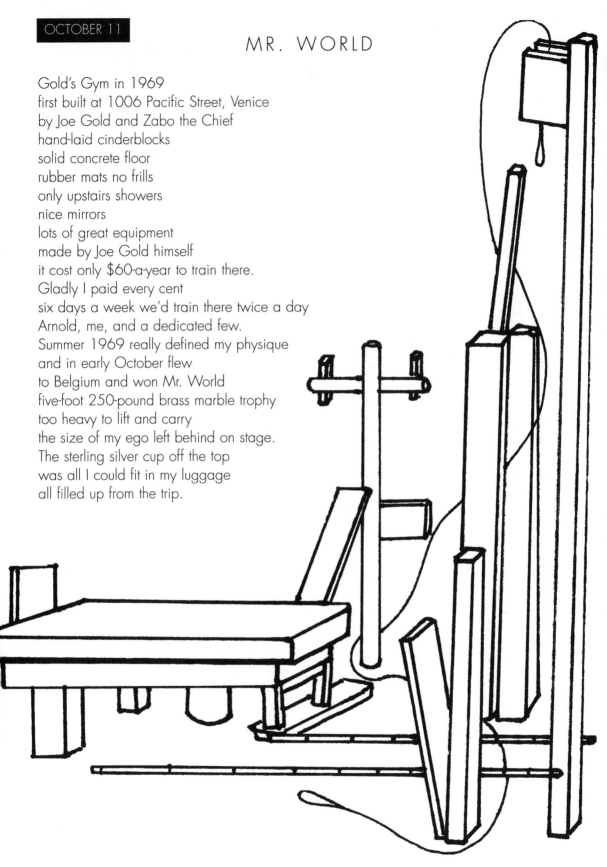

Gold's Gym in 1969
first built at 1006 Pacific Street, Venice
by Joe Gold and Zabo the Chief
hand-laid cinderblocks
solid concrete floor
rubber mats no frills
only upstairs showers
nice mirrors
lots of great equipment
made by Joe Gold himself
it cost only $60-a-year to train there.
Gladly I paid every cent
six days a week we'd train there twice a day
Arnold, me, and a dedicated few.
Summer 1969 really defined my physique
and in early October flew
to Belgium and won Mr. World
five-foot 250-pound brass marble trophy
too heavy to lift and carry
the size of my ego left behind on stage.
The sterling silver cup off the top
was all I could fit in my luggage
all filled up from the trip.

WORKOUT 148

My heaviest squatting day ever came training with Arnold five weeks before the 1972 Mr. Universe contest in London. Here's what we did in late August at Gold's Gym, Pacific Street, Venice. The next day my lower back and right knee were really sore.

leg extensions
two sets of 12 reps
one-leg back stretch
leg curl
two sets of 12 reps
squats
135, 185, 225, 285, 315, 365, and 405 pounds for 10 reps (Arnold did same weights but with eight reps on his last set)
leg extensions
three sets of 10 reps
leg curl
three sets of 10 reps
leg press
three sets of 10 reps
hack squats
three sets of 10 reps

CALVES
donkeys (each other on lower back)
holding 50-pound plate for five sets of 20 reps
standing calf raise
three sets of 15 reps with heavy weight
seated calf raise
three sets of 15 reps with 125 pounds (Arnold used more)

ABS
crunches
100 reps
leg raises
100 reps
twists
100 reps

OLD MUSCLE BEACH

Artie Zeller
great photographer storyteller
with his camera captured memories
frozen moments that live forever.
Told me story of Buick Hotel
on Speedway right near the beach
bodybuilder slept in back seat of '53 Buick
abandoned under street light
showered at the gym
for breakfast stole only one quart of milk
read late at night
his best interests served rent free
until the city turned off electricity.

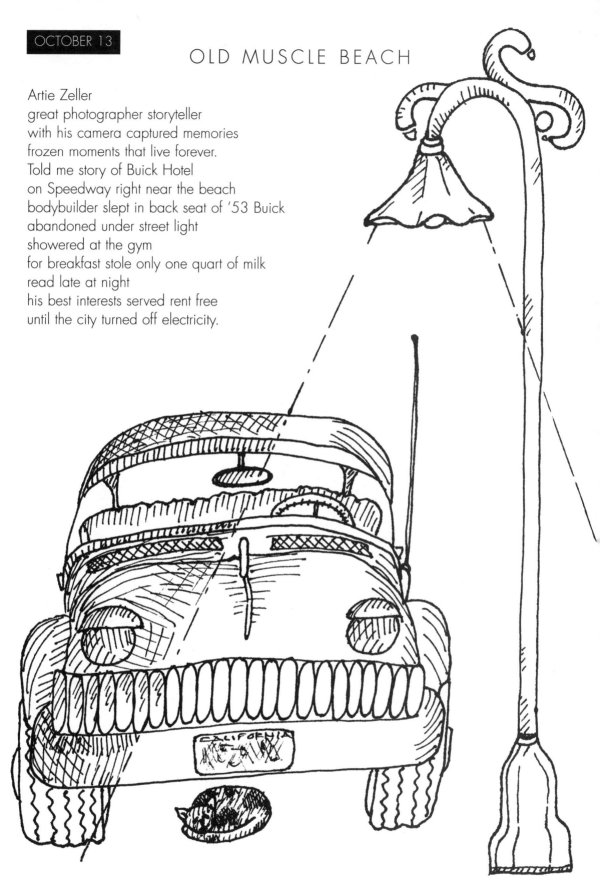

WORKOUT 149

I did *delts-arms* training for the 1970 Mr. Universe in London. Arnold was preparing for his first Olympia win, and Dave Draper and Franco Colombu were in the gym.

WARM-UP
barbell cleans and press
two sets of 12 reps, then moving down the dumbbell rack did the following nonstop sets:

DELTS
dumbbell presses
60, 55, 50, 45, 40, and 35 pounds for eight to 10 reps (after a few minutes rest did it again, then again)
press behind neck
a few sets at 135 pounds for 10 reps
dumbbell side raises
25, 30, and 35 pounds for 10 reps
one-arm side raises
three nonstop sets of 12 reps with 20 pounds each arm
bent over rear delt cable raises
three sets of 12 reps with 25 pounds

ARMS
{ dumbbell concentration curl
35, 40, 45, and 50 pounds for 10 reps
{ one-arm dumbbell extension
35, 40, 45, and 50 pounds for 10 reps
{ 45-degree incline dumbbell curl
four sets of 10 reps with 35 pounds
{ triceps pressdown on lat machine
four sets of 10 reps (Arnold's arms were huge, pumped and round)

FOREARMS
barbell reverse curl
three sets of 10 reps with 80 pounds
barbell wrist curl
three sets of 10 reps with 135 pounds

ABS
crunches
100 reps
leg raises
100 reps
seated twist
100 reps

THE TRICKSTER

Ode to Arnold
evolved trickster archetype
flies in private jet planes
rides in long white limousines
black tie show business charity events

negotiation intelligence
20 million dollar movies out of sight
all the money he made and spent
while I write
to pay the summer rent.

WORKOUT 150

Itrained for Mr. America during the summer of 1968 in my St. Petersburg, Florida, home gym (200 square feet adjacent to patio pool) for six days a week with simple equipment: dumbbells, preacher bench, barbell, squat rack, dip bars, lat machine, crude leg curl/extension. I did a two-way split routine: Day One: *back, biceps, forearms, thighs, calves*; Day Two: *chest, shoulders, triceps, abs*. I also trained at Harry Smith's gym 20 miles away in Tampa.

BACK
front pulldown
three sets of 10 reps
T-bar row
three sets of 10 reps
one-arm cable row
three sets of 10 reps each arm

BICEPS
alternate dumbbell curl
three sets of 10 reps
preacher bench curl (heavy weight with EZ curl bar)
three sets of 10 reps

FOREARMS
barbell reverse curl
three sets of 15 reps
wrist curl (with Olympic bar)
135 pounds for three sets of 15 reps

THIGH
leg curl
three sets of 10 reps
leg extension
three sets of 10 reps
squats
four sets for eight to 10 reps working up to 375 pounds
stiff-legged deadlift
three sets of 10 reps to stretch hamstrings

CALVES
standing calf raise
four sets of 15 reps
seated calf raise
four sets of 15 reps

JOE WEIDER

Joe Weider
bodybuilding leader 50 years
taught Arnold much of what he knows
always generous with advice
wants to know

how I like this month's Muscle & Fitness.
If it weren't for Joe
bodybuilding wouldn't be where it is today
he gave everybody
free publicity.

OCTOBER 18

W O R K O U T   1 5 1

In the fall of 1968, I found myself teaching math in Tarpon Springs, Florida, in an old junior high school. It was so hot in September that the only place I could cool off was during my daily air conditioned hour-drive on Interstate 19 in my 1965 Chevy Nova. I couldn't wait to get home, float in my pool, eat, and begin three hours of heavy *chest-shoulder-triceps* training. Today, I'd use lighter weights and slower negatives with less rest between sets.

CHEST
bench press (bouncing out reps)
  five or six sets working up to 10 reps with 300
  pounds
incline dumbbell press
  five sets of eight to 10 reps ending with 110-pound
  dumbbells
parallel dips (with added weight around my
waist)
  four sets of eight to 10 reps up to 150 pounds
dumbbell fly
  four sets of 10 reps ending with 70 pounders
dumbbell pullover across bench
  four sets of 10 reps ending with 100-pound dumbbell

DELTS
press behind neck
  up to 200 pounds for eight reps on my fourth set
dumbbell side raises
  four sets of 10 reps up to 40 pounders
bent over dumbbell rear delt raises
  four sets of 10 reps with 25-pound weights

TRICEPS
pressdown
  five sets of 10 reps
one-arm dumbbell extension
  three sets of 10 reps
reverse triceps dip
  three sets of 20 reps with no weight

ABS
Roman chair situps
  200 reps
leg raises (on flat bench)
  four sets of 50 reps
seated twists
  200 reps

BACK IN PRESENT TIME

Awoke to a cool 50-degree 5:00 A.M. morning
listened to harmonica music I just recorded
I called Bach wards and Forewards
on my sound table
covered myself with a sheepskin
heard sound with my whole body
resonance reverberation
after 50 minutes
created a delightful sensation
all through my muscle and bones
frequency following response
sight sound vibration massage
lock on to powerful frequency
of Bach backwards.
I have done a lot of light sound entrainment
over the last 10 years so that now
when I just listen to music
I see and feel its shape and size
as the musical body
begins to materialize.

OCTOBER 20

GURU'S THREE-FOOT VERTICAL JUMP

Sri Chinmoy soars to new heights
leaps straight up high into the air
grasshoppers, kangaroos, bullfrogs beware
stratosphere prepare
it's scary up there
be wary of the step
right at the top
of the vertical stair
where 4 by 6 by 24 inch
wooden blocks stacked
up
will take care
of muscle wear and tear
creating an atmosphere
of fearlessness rare
to see, hear, and share
inspiring all found
still hanging around
way down on the ground.

WORKOUT 152

The year 1965 was the beginning of my real competitive bodybuilding career. During the summer I was going to Old Dominion College in Virginia Beach four nights a week studying geology and astronomy. I trained with Jim Haislop at the American Health Club in Norfolk six days a week starting at 10 A.M. after a breakfast of one dozen soft boiled eggs and a quart of orange juice. We did the old Ironman routine which Haislop said had worked well for him with his calves like Steve Reeves. I learned that you must take your calf exercises to a burn in order to grow. I did *back-biceps-forearms-thighs-calves* on Monday, Wednesday, Friday; and *chest-shoulders-triceps* on Tuesday, Thursday, Saturday. I remember a typical summer day when we did

front chin
three sets of 10 reps
pulldown behind neck
three sets of 10 with 200 pounds
T-bar row
three 45-pound plates at the end, three sets of 10 reps
one-arm dumbbell row
100 pounds for three sets of 10 reps

BICEPS
alternate dumbbell curl
50 pounds for three sets of 10 reps
one-arm dumbbell concentration curl
40 pounds for three sets of 10 reps
incline dumbbell curl
35 pounds for three sets of 10 reps

FOREARMS
reverse curl
100-pound barbell for three sets of 10 reps
wrist curl
three sets of 15 reps with 135 pounds

LEGS
squats
135, 185, 225, 275, 315, 355 pounds for 10 reps
leg extension
three sets of 10 reps
leg curl
three sets of 10 reps with a comfortable weight
standing calf raises
15 reps alternating each leg like in a walking motion, then did reps with both legs simultaneously to an extreme burn

ABS
flat bench leg raise
four sets of 25 reps
Roman chair situps
100 nonstop reps
seated twists
100 reps

DREAM OF THE WALL

Dreaming, built a wall
all around myself
muscles hold this wall
in place on the surface
at my face
level outside body boundaries.
It's the room
created by body's extension
my dynamic sphere
appendages in all directions
it's the meaning in the expression
keep your distance.
This room of myself
I live in could be bigger
expand 3-D boundaries
smash into infinite space all around.
In a way only space exists
matter is dense atmosphere.
This Wall symbolizes the boundaries of my Heart cave
where dreaming I crawled in through tunnel
into chamber of self inside and there was the
Golden Monarch Butterfly
huge wide wing taps my head
as if to say
wake up
this is it
take a look
here I am
your guardian angel
can fly anywhere
but dwells here
perpetually all times of year.

WORKOUT 153

During a hot muggy summer in August of 1965 in Norfolk, Virginia, I did a *chest-shoulder-triceps* workout. After the workout, I drove around in my misty green 1958 Chevy to the Giant Supermarket where I bought a two-pound thick T-bone steak. For 50 cents more, they grilled it medium rare and I ate it with a baked potato. That summer my bodyweight shot up from 185 to 205 pounds from all the heavy training and eating.

CHEST

bench press with a very wide grip
working up to 295 pounds for 10 reps (it wasn't long before my shoulders began to hurt from the stress of that wide grip, so I switched to a shoulder-width grip instead which led to dropping my poundages)

45-degree incline dumbbell press
three sets of 10 reps with 115-pound dumbbells

dumbbell fly
50, 60, and 70 pounds for 10 reps each set

dumbbell pullover across bench
90, 100, and 110 pounds for 10 reps

seated dumbbell front press
three sets of 10 reps with 70 pounds

dumbbell side raises
40, 45, and 50 pounds for 10 reps

bent over rear delt raises
25, 30, and 35 pounds for 10 reps

dumbbell upright row
three sets of 10 reps with 50 pounders

TRICEPS

pressdown
90 pounds for three sets of 10 reps

lying triceps extension
three sets of 10 reps with 100 pounds

one-arm dumbbell kickback
three sets of 10 reps with 30 pounds

ABS

{ **leg raise** (on flat bench)
Roman chair situp
both four sets of 25 reps

seated twist
100 reps

hyperextension
two sets of 15 reps

1968 MR. AMERICA AND MR. UNIVERSE

Nineteen sixty-eight was the first year I began to make my mark in bodybuilding:
first winning IFBB Mr. America in New York
and the very next week Mr. Universe in Miami
beating Arnold that day became
my claim to fame.
People ask how it felt but must admit
I already knew I'd win for Jim Haislop did compete
with him the week before in London
told me Arnold not yet near his peak
sure made up for it subsequent years of his career.

BIG TREES OF PALM SPRINGS

Eucalyptus trees gigantic roots
life network shoots
inside acres of Mother Earth
around my home a stable foundation
shock absorber for land gyration.
Mighty trunk ten feet thick
grows huge branches that stick
up hundreds of feet.
The cool wind frees
bark and 10,000 leaves
dancing as they land
in late afternoon.
Venus and a crescent moon
glisten in the western sky
and across the galaxy fly
in the desert.
I don't ask why
as daylight fades.
Soon it will be dark.

WORKOUT 154

Living and teaching school in New Jersey 1965-66
won twenty trophies in one year
height class Mr. Universe, Mr. Eastern America
Mr. North America and lots of bodypart awards, best legs, best poser
remember training in the garage of the house where I was staying
in winter 20 degrees in gloves and overcoat below freezing, it was hard to
get a good pump
so started training in school locker room, kept my weights
locked in a trunk, had everything I needed for heavy workouts.
One day worked legs and after five sets of heavy calf raises
with a wooden machine I'd made attached to the wall
I did three sets of 20 reps in the full squat with 325 pounds
collapsing after each set breathless on the floor
after 10 minutes got up and did more
also did three sets of hacks holding 35-pound dumbbells for 10 reps
and stiff-legged deadlift 100 pounds three sets of 10
then drove to where I lived in my light blue
new 1966 Mustang, opened the door, stepped out
stood up, legs cramped, collapsed
lay there a half hour before I could move
got up, my rest period had lapsed
thought it was time for my next set of squats.

SOUND OF LIGHT

Since in the beginning
was the word
with light yet unborn
not seen, only heard.
Morning meditation
began after a brisk walk
with Tyler around the block
a look at the clock
told me it was 6 A.M. sharp
and time for meditation.
Listening to blues harp

bright music recorded reverbed
closed my eyes
light was all I heard
enlightened brilliance seen
without wearing glasses
of my Mind-Muscle machine.
Some kind of learning had taken place
enabling me to see the sounds of
music
without red L.E.D.s blinking in front of
my face.

W O R K O U T   1 5 5

During the winter of 1965, I worked out in a New Jersey garage wearing sweat pants, two T-shirts, a sweat jersey, gloves (I found it hard to hold a cold dumbbell without them), a scarf, and an overcoat. I could see my breath so I did the training with little rest between sets to avoid freezing. All I had were three pairs of adjustable dumbbells and an adjustable incline bench. I did *chest-shoulders-triceps*:

incline dumbbell press
   three sets of 10 reps with 90, 100, and 110 pounds
dumbbell fly
   three sets of 10 reps with 60, 65,and 70 pounds
dumbbell pullover
   three sets of 10 reps with 100 pounds
seated dumbbell press
   10 reps with 55, 60, and 65 pounds
dumbbell side raises
   12 reps with 30, 35, and 40 pounds
bent over dumbbell rear delt raises
   three sets of 12 reps with 25 pounds
seated triceps extension
   three sets of 10 reps while holding a 90-pound dumbbell with two hands
one-arm seated triceps extension
   three sets of 10 reps with 40 pounds
dumbbell kickback
   three sets of 12 reps with 30 pounds
{ **leg raise**
  crunches
   both three sets of 30 reps

DREAM BODY

Watching the light
evoked by music
that is bright
visualizing the dream body
I see a symbol
from my only painting
created after hearing for the first time
Mozart Piano Concerto 19

a heart with wings
outlines the feeling of the body
I wear when I travel in dreams
eyes-closed mock-ups
goal-oriented fantasies
projects me anywhere in the universe
I want to be.

WORKOUT 156

In the summer of 1964, I was just out of college and looking for a teaching job in Pennsylvania. I found it in Hamburg. I taught six classes a day of algebra, geometry, trigonometry—a lot of lonely work for only $4500 a year. I formed a bodybuilding club with 4000 pounds of weights donated by the local iron foundry. Some kids in the club built a lat machine, and I brought in lots of muscle magazines. After school one day, I did the following *back-biceps-forearms* workout finishing by 5 P.M., then drove my '57 Plymouth 20 miles south to my home in Reading, PA above a health studio.

front pulldown
170, 180, and 190 pounds for 10 reps
T-bar row
130, 140, and 150 pounds for 10 reps
one-arm dumbbell row
90 pounds for three sets of 10 reps with one-arm lat stretch
shrugs
three sets of 12 reps with 100 pound dumbbells

BICEPS
alternate dumbbell curls
40, 45, and 50 pounds for 10 reps
one-arm dumbbell concentration curl
three nonstop sets of 10 reps with 35 pounds
incline dumbbell curl
35 pounds for 10 reps, 40 for nine, 40 for eight

FOREARMS
barbell reverse curl
90, 100, and 110 pounds for 10 reps
barbell wrist curl
three sets of 15 reps with 135 pounds

ABS
leg raise
four sets of 25 reps
Roman chair situps
100 reps
seated twists
100 reps
hyperextension
two sets of 20 reps

NUTRITION IN THE 1960S

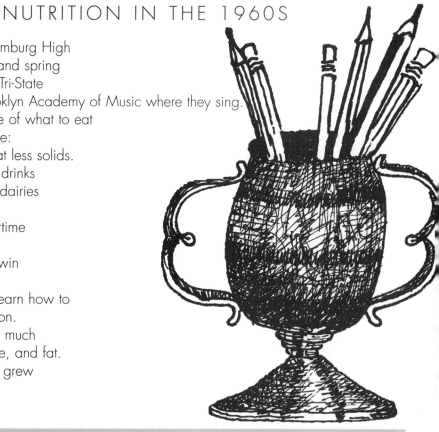

After teaching at Hamburg High
through fall, winter, and spring
trained for IFBB Mr. Tri-State
in New York at Brooklyn Academy of Music where they sing.
With little experience of what to eat
my theory was simple:
drink more liquids eat less solids.
drank lots of protein drinks
Raw milk from local dairies
Soy protein powder
blender worked overtime
all the time.
No wonder I didn't win
but I placed
took me a while to learn how to
lose fat build definition.
It was all about how much
protein, carbohydrate, and fat.
My trophy collection grew
once I learned that.

WORKOUT 157

During my senior year in college I slept on massage table at Figure Tone Health Studio in Wilkes-Barre, Pa. I got up early, made breakfast, walked to class everyday. In my '53 Dodge, I drove home, took a nap, studied until 9 P.M., then drove back to health studio where I trained with big bulked-up manager who sold memberships to women who couldn't say no. One evening we did the following quick-paced moderate weights leg workout, and afterwards my legs went numb for the first time.

leg extension
five sets of 10 reps
leg press
five sets of 10 reps
hack squat
five sets of 10 reps
leg curl
five sets of 10 reps
donkey calf raises
10 sets of 20 reps
{ **leg raise**
four sets of 50 reps
Roman chair situps
four sets of 50 reps
seated twist
four sets of 50 reps

OUT OF MY MIND

The first time that it happened
was in chem lab, an experiment called gravimetric analysis
understood procedure got so involved
forgot I was me
doing chemistry
in present time
my self that was mine
became the same as the task at hand.
Felt like I worked 9 A.M. until noon
look outside not what I planned
instead saw the moon.
Immediately I knew
my attention was me and got an A
that day time flew
in chemistry
laboratory.

1963 MR. KEYSTONE STATE

During my junior year in college I finally began enjoying workout freedom
after switching my major from chemistry to education
I'd won some time for serious training
and got back into shape after two years of brain exhaustion
from calculus, physics, qualitative and quantitative analysis
and now I could enjoy liberal arts and bodybuilding.
Trained at Bob Ceccoli's home gym in the basement
behind his drive-in restaurant called the "Victory Pig" in Forty Fort.
People came from miles around to taste his secret pizza recipe
and I'd drive there after class to work out.
There was my friend Hal Raker who deadlifted 525 at 132-pound bodyweight
we drove all over Pennsylvania in his 1958 Chevy Impala on weekends
to see all the weight-lifting and physique competitions and
one weekend our local group organized the Mr. Keystone State in Kingston.
Came in second lifting in the 181-pound class weighing 168
with a 165-pound curl, 275-pound bench press, and 425-pound deadlift
and won the physique competition with Bob coming in third.
After that, gained a little respect from the gym heavyweight
Big Otto who bench pressed 400 pounds and owned a bar in Duryea.
He was his own bouncer. His hands were weapons he shaped as he chuckled
hitting his middle knuckle hundreds of reps every day with a hammer.
His victims got the point that he didn't need brass knuckles.
Remember showing Otto my new posing trunks before the show.
He said why don't you wait until you get the body first.
But there was no time to wait in my mind I know.

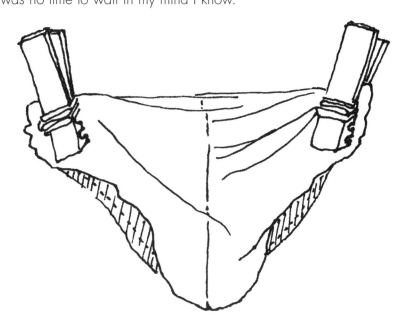

WORKOUT 158

In the days before formal organized split routine training, I sometimes worked my whole body in one day especially when training for powerlifting or "odd lifting" as it was called then since the lifts were different from the three Olympic lifts. I had wished they would include the squat in our contest because I was a good squatter even then and no doubt could have squatted 400 pounds or more for one rep. I had always done sets of 10 reps with at least 300 pounds, but that wasn't about being a good deadlifter. Here's my last workout before the Mr. Keystone State meet:

Olympic bar curl
65 pounds for 10 reps, 95 for six, 115 for three, then one rep with 135, 145, and 155 pounds without cheating or excess swinging

bench press
135 pounds for 10 reps, 165 for six, 195 for three, then one rep with 225, 245, 255, and 265 pounds

deadlift
135 pounds for 10 reps, 185 for six, 225 for five, 275 for three, then one rep with 315, 355, 380, and 400 pounds, this was the most I ever did prior to the meet

But that night in front of the audience I discovered a power inside me that made me stronger. Confident, I made all three attempts on each lift: curl 145, 155, 165 pounds; bench press 255, 265, 275 pounds; and deadlift 375 pounds, then 400 went up easy. I knew I couldn't win first but I was a sure second. So I took 425 pounds for my final deadlift attempt and it went up so easily I said to myself, "I can't believe how strong I am today." Happy with a second place finish, I went back to my regular pace of studying and training but hurt my lower back in deadlift training six month later. Consequently, I lost my ambition and bombed out in bench press in a YMCA contest. After that I concentrated on bodybuilding competition.

MY FIRST
BODYBUILDING CONTEST

My Open Novice 1961, Emmaus, PA.
It was springtime and I was 18
a freshman in college still not bogged down in studying
as reflected in my low grades, but my training was keen
and I came well prepared for my first competition
with my posing routine down cold.
How could I forget four poses?
Front double biceps, side triceps, rear lat spread and overhead shot told
the judges I deserved attention and fifth place was what I got.
Not bad out of 45 contestants I said to myself but
the real compliment came from Bob Hoffman himself
famous father of American weight-lifting
watching me back stage pumping up actually said to me
"If I had your physique
I'd walk around all day with my shirt off."
After that knew I had a great future in bodybuilding to seek.

MY SECOND
BODYBUILDING COMPETITION

One month later I was back in Emmaus again to compete
this time for Mr. Pennsylvania title.
This was the big time and after watching the heavyweights complete
their last clean and jerk around midnight
went back stage to change and pump-up for the physique meet
stood with 12 glistening bodies in front of the black curtain draped
hanging from a basketball hoop, then it all went so fast
thought I might get sixth or seventh place
but came in dead last
because I wasn't a weight lifter and scored no points for athletic ability
even though I was a good archer I had no proof.
Bill March won Mr. Pennsylvania
and he also won the 198-pound weightlifting that evening.
After the show I congratulated him and asked if he remembered me
since I met him at the last meet, but to him I was just another admiring fan
without a face
in last place.

WORKOUT 159

I was too naive to be discouraged. Finishing last fueled my training for the 1961 Teen Age Mr. America being held in York, PA. Though at 18 I had another year left in this contest but I was going to do my best to win it this year. I already had the posing trunks and the posing routine down cold so I could feel confident about winning. I trained hard at the Wilkes Barre YMCA and Bob's Gym with a two-day split routine: Day One was upper body, and Day Two was legs, abs, and basketball. It was the end of my freshman year and I worked at Wilkes College library for a salary of 75 cents an hour. It felt as if I were working for free but I scrimped and saved my money for a bus trip to York and placed third that day— winning my first bodybuilding trophy. Here's what I did in my upper body training at the YMCA on June 3, 1961.

bench press
135 pounds for 10 reps, 185 for eight, 225 for six
front chin
three sets of 10 reps with a wide grip
dumbbell pullover
75 pounds for 3 sets of 10 reps
dumbbell flyes
three sets of 10 reps with 40 pounders
barbell clean
100 pounds for 10 reps, 120 for eight, 140 for six
front press
100 pounds for 10 reps, 120 for eight, 140 for six
dumbbell side raises
three sets of 10 reps with 35 pounds
bent over rowing
100 pounds for 10 reps, 120 for eight, 140 for six
reverse dips
three sets of 10 reps with a 45-pound plate on my lap, feet on a bench straight out in front of me
barbell curl
100 pounds for three sets of 10 reps
wrist curl
100 pounds for three sets of 10 reps

WORKOUT 160

I was training six days a week for the Teen Age Mr. America contest. The next day was Day Two of my split routine, so I worked legs and abs at Bob's Gym, which had a leg curl and leg extension machine I had not seen at the YMCA. Afterwards, I drove home, ate, read, relaxed a bit, then hitch-hiked to the Y where I sunbathed from 1 to 3 P.M. up on the sunroof. Then I checked out a basketball and played full court basketball solitaire in the gym, dribbling and shooting hoops, thinking that all I can do is win.

squats
135, 185, 225, 275, and 315 pounds for 10 reps
leg extension
three sets of 10 reps
leg curl
three sets of 10 reps
standing calf raises (on the calf machine)
six sets of 15 reps
donkeys (with a 200-pound rider)
four sets of 15 reps
Roman chair situps
100 reps
leg raises
four sets of 25 reps

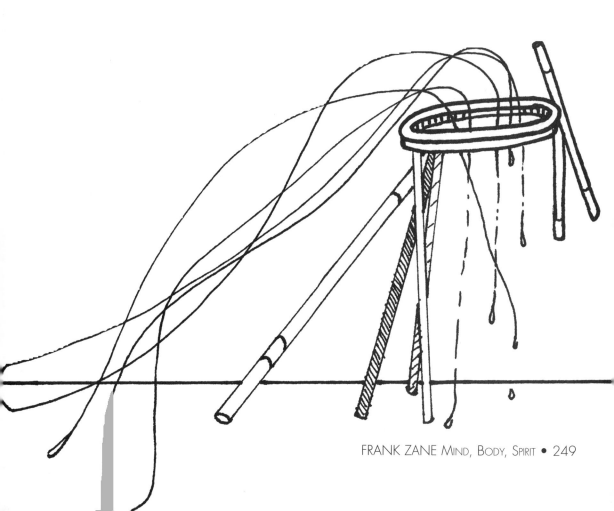

TEEN AGE MR. AMERICA

The Greyhound bus arrived in York, PA.
early morning that warm June day
I was tanned and in shape
weighing 168 with a 27-inch waist
wasted no time changing into my white posing trunks
pumping up feels great
I thought as I hit the weights for the last time before we went on stage.
Before I knew I was feeling a charge from placing third
winning my first bodybuilding trophy.
First place Steve Boyer of Carlisle, PA.
was amazing at five-foot eight
with his 19-inch arms he looked great
and Nick Spano of Atlanta, GA. both were 19, it was their last year
and everybody expected me to win the next year. I couldn't wait.
But by the following year, my focus had changed.
Sophomore year as a chemistry major working two jobs
left me little time to train, spending all day in chem lab
keeping flab off my body wasn't easy with little training
and a diet less than strict. That summer before the contest
got a job as a waiter at a Pocono resort where starchy food on my plate
1962 Teen Age Mr. America ninth place led to verdict.
Depressed, cursed my fate in a York bar, drank beer waiting
for my bus back to the Poconos. During the long night ride
thought "Now I know not to brag ahead of time."

My earliest recorded workout comes from my 1959 diary. I spent the summer before my senior year in high school as an archery instructor at Camp Acahela Boy Scout camp in Blakeslee, PA. Because of a lot of practice, I could hit the 6-inch bullseye every time at 30 yards with my 50-pound pull Root recurve bow shooting aluminum arrows. On alternate days, I'd practice kicking a football loaned to me by Coach Cimakasky with my cleated shoes. I was able to get off 80-yard long spirals which seemed to assure my place as punter on Edwardsville High School football team. I built my bodyweight up to 160 pounds by drinking lots of milk. This was were I ate and stayed, training with my one-dumbbell gym kept by my bed in the bunkhouse under my bench. On weekends, I'd hitchhike 25 miles to home carrying my 55-pound gym in a pillow case. I worked out three days a week with the following routine:

one-legged squats
  three sets of 10 reps holding a 25 pound dumbbell in one hand, standing on a bench with one leg

one-legged calf raises
  three sets of 15 reps

sissy squat
  no weight for three sets of 20 reps

one-arm dumbbell row
  55 pounds three sets of 10 reps

good morning exercise
  same weight on my back

one-arm press
  three sets of 10 reps with 45, 50, and 55 pounds

dumbbell pullover (lying across the bench)
  three sets of 10 reps with 55 pounds

one arm rubber cable crossover
  with one end of my cable attached to the knob on a door

21 curl with a swingbell (a dumbbell bar with all the plates it the middle)
  three sets with 30 pounds, seven reps from bottom to half way, seven reps from half way to top, then seven full reps

one-arm dumbbell extension
  three sets of 10 reps with 25 pounds

{ **half situps**
  leg raises
  both three sets of 25 reps

seated twists
  100 reps with a pole on my shoulders

skipped rope for 5 minutes

I LIVE MY LIFE BY DREAMS

These diaries wouldn't be complete
without relating a recurrent dream
I've always had before competition
which told me exactly when to start training
   hard:
I'm at a bodybuilding contest wearing a
   long overcoat
no one recognizes me, I need a haircut and
   a shave
and so does my body, so I remove my
   clothes
and start shaving and after I remove the
   hair
I discover there's little muscle there
nothing but white skin, extra bodyfat
now they're calling me on stage
skinny and smooth, muscles look flat
can't find my trunks, don't even look good
   for my age
wake up and realize that
I'd better start training hard now
before it's too late.

MY EARLIEST
PRODUCTIVE WORKOUTS

After doing a little bodybuilding at the YMCA
got a job as a pinboy in ninth grade when I was 14
saved my money and at the end of the school year
had $275 so signed up to go
to Philmont Scout Ranch in Cimarron, New Mexico.
Five-day bus ride there, five days back
ten days hiking, horseback riding
nighttime campfire singing songs playing harmonica
one night a long 100-pound log with grips at each end
lay waiting for lifting.
Twenty-five explorer scouts attempted to lift it overhead
only one succeeded and it wasn't me
promised myself I would
build myself up
when I got home, so I got a pinboy job at the JCC
and bought a pair of adjustable 15-pound dumbbells
and began training in my basement after school
six days a week, upper body one day, legs the next
during my sophomore year in high school.
My father was mad, I should have been cutting the grass but
I saw my muscles look my best
with lats sticking out after only two weeks
I resolved to continue training hard to
build a quality physique.

WORKOUT 162

Aside from my new dumbbell set, I accumulated other equipment: 20-pound solid iron railroad car wheels, 30-pound large iron pulley wheel, and flywheels from an auto junkyard. They all fit on a six-foot iron bar placed on a wooden squat rack. On a typical day I'd do

bench press
three sets of 10 reps
wide-grip top deadlift (from the bench)
pullover with swingbell (lying across a giant curved log)
stretched my ribcage and gave me foundation to develop great serratus
flies and pullover combination
(around-the-world dumbbell exercise) three sets of 10 reps
dumbbell side raise
three sets of 10 reps
seated dumbbell curl
three sets of 10 reps
kickbacks
three sets of 10 reps

LEGS
squats
three sets of 10 reps working up to 300 pounds
stiff-legged deadlift
a few sets for hamstrings
donkey calf raise
three sets of 15 reps (sitting on my back was my brother Adam, who had inherited my mother's great calves)

ABS
situps
100 reps
leg raise
100 reps
seated twist
100 reps

GREAT UNCLE JOHN

Uncle John bum of my youth passed away long ago
just where when how
I don't know.
He'd appear every now and then
when the weather was warm
sacks of blueberries from Larksville mountain on each arm
for us in exchange for a hot meal and bath
a few dollars for wine then he'd disappear
until we saw him again with blueberries this time
when the weather was warm again next year.

WORKOUT 163

I began doing Hatha Yoga at age 16. I would get up early each morning and assume the postures, stretching, relaxing, and breathing deep. Then I'd sit in a lotus posture upright and master the Pranayama breath control exercise, then meditate on breathing watching the flow of my thinking. All this took a half hour. I'd eat and a little later go running in Larksville Mountain. I'd run up, run across the top, run down—six miles in all. By the fall I was doing it quickly not even taxing my breathing. Some people wondered why I ran when I wasn't even going out for football. At least I was getting into the altered state caused by endorphin release. It got to the point that I could keep running and not become fatigued. I had so much endurance that it was scary . . . so I stopped. I got more into weight training with my simple routine using dumbbells, a barbell, and a bench.

clean and overhead dumbbell press
  two sets of 10 reps
barbell row
  two sets of 10 reps
close grip bench press
  two sets of 10 reps
dumbbell side raises
  two sets of 10 reps
alternate dumbbell curl
  two sets of 10 reps
dumbbell kickback
  two sets of 10 reps
barbell reverse curl
  two sets of 10 reps
barbell front squat
  two sets of 10 reps
one-legged calf raise
  two sets of 15 reps
{ **leg raise**
  crunches
    both two sets of 30 reps
seated twist
  100 reps

DICHOTOMIES

No life without death
no growth without damage
no mending without breaking
no theft without the taking
no construction without destruction
no spending without earning

no learning without the yearning
no living without the liver
no giving without the giver
no money without the business
no being without the is-ness
no exit without existence.

WORKOUT 164

The most radical *abs* workouts I ever had were in 1970 training at Gold's Gym when
I began doing
Roman chair situps longer and longer. With a mental exercise to occupy my mind,
I closed my eyes
and started doing situps. Focusing my attention in the four upper corners of the room,
I visualized
myself doing situps below from this vantage point. I'd hold this scenario until all images
faded,
then I'd visualize myself as a white-winged red heart with a golden triangle in the center
and fly
anywhere I wished. My first abdominal trip lasted one hour and aside from lower back
stiffness the
next day—along with sore abs—I had the feeling I could do more. One day Arnold
walked in amidst
one of my situp trances and claimed he tried to talk to me. He got no response. Even
Arnold
couldn't distract me that day. Over the next week I pushed my ab trip to two and a half
hours and at
the end I knew I could just keep going. So I stopped.

WORKOUT 165

Elastics is the name of a training system
using dumbbells and rubber cables simultaneously
each exercise at the same time
with dumbbell in hand holding cable, too
the other end of the cable
is under your shoe
and in this position
there are many exercise you can do
here are a few:
using two five-pound dumbbells and two rubber cables, too
I like one set of 20 reps each exercise
move slowly and do
isometric stops tensing near the top
and on the way down slow negatives and stops:
overhead press, side lateral raise, front chest pulls, curls, kickbacks
and doorway stretch is a quick session
less than 10 minutes that will
maintain upper body definition.

MILL VALLEY 1978

Mike Murphy co-founder of Esalen Institute
remember when I went to see
him and Aikido master George Leonard to boot
in Mill Valley 1978, Ken O'Neill and me.
Lifted weights then ran four miles
if memory serves me we weren't even tired.
They were amazed at my color slides
showing before and after physical transformations.
Since then Mike's written *The Future of the Body*:
"The soul or spirit has boundaries, unique form, a point of view
location which can move in some sort of environment
and continuity with its life upon earth . . .
The (soul) vehicle of survival even has a face and organs . . .
a conscious self, or person, that inhabits particular locations in the spirit world.
It sometimes encounters other spirits, views marvelous or terrible soulscapes,
hears unearthly music, touches other forms and has intercourse with them,
moves from place to place, and acts upon its environment.
Such descriptions indicate that this traveling self,
this soul is a kind of body.
Indeed, there may be a fundamental equation
between personhood and embodiment,
in this world or any other."

WORKOUT 166

Using light weights for a quick one set of 10 to 15 rhythmic reps with slow negatives, I'd pump up my muscle memory to reactivate the more dormant neuro-muscular pathways. Between the following exercises, I'd do two- or one-arm lat stretches for 15 seconds:

front pulldown
150 pounds for 12 reps
cable crossover behind neck
40 pounds for 15 reps
low cable row
140 pounds for 12 reps
reverse pec deck
55 pounds for 12 reps
close grip pulldown
140 pounds for 12 reps
dumbbell shrug
55 pounds for 12 reps
one-arm dumbbell row
70 pounds for 12 reps
pronated arms back stretch between sets of exercises

BICEPS
one-arm dumbbell concentration curl
30 pounds for 12 reps
alternate dumbbell curl
30 pounds for 12 reps
face down incline dumbbell curl
25 pounds for 15 reps
preacher cable curl
70 pounds for 12 reps

FOREARMS
barbell reverse wrist curl
35 pounds for 12 reps
barbell wrist curl
50 pounds for 20 reps
gripper
15 reps, shook out my hands so it would be easier to do

ABS
hanging knee-ups
30 reps
crunches
30 reps
one-arm cable curl
70 pounds for 20 reps each arm
hyperextension
20 reps

VAST MIND

Vast space is perfect
the middle way
not too much or too little
judging, accepting, rejecting
we miss the true nature of things.

Neither living in entanglement
nor in inner empty feelings
the oneness of things is what it all means
just let all and everything be as it is
being thus, I pass through the strife on the
nature of life.

WORKOUT 167

To keep a trim waistline, I prioritize abs by working them first before lunch, followed by a leg workout. The only rest I'd take would be to enhance my flexibility between the leg exercises and to do stretches with one-leg back and one-leg up. Afterwards, perspiring profusely, I was hardly able to walk—thank God it wasn't hot outside.

ABS
hanging knee-ups
25 reps
crunches
35 reps
one-arm cable crunches
20 reps with 70 pounds
seated twist
50 reps
incline leg raise
30 reps
two-arm cable crunch
20 reps with 80 pounds
hyperextensions
20 reps

LEGS
leg extension
120 pounds for 12 reps
leg curl
70 pounds for 12 reps
leg press
180 pounds for 12 reps
Leg Blaster squat
135 pounds for 10 reps
hip machine
90 pounds 12 reps
standing one legged curl
40 pounds for 12 reps
standing calf raise (with my Leg Blaster)
135 pounds for 20 reps, holding 5 seconds at the top
hot burn
leg press calf raises
15 reps with 180 pounds
seated calf raise
80 pounds for 15 reps
donkey calf machine
15 reps with 220 pounds

MATTHEW 6:26, 28-29, 7:7-9

Look at the wild birds;
they sow not, they reap not
they gather nothing in granaries
and yet your heavenly Father feeds them.
Look how the lilies of the field grow;
they neither toil not spin
and yet, I tell you even King Solomon
in all his grandeur was never robed like any one of them.
Ask and the gift will be yours
seek and you will find
knock and the door will open to you
for everyone who asks receives
the seeker finds
the door is open to anyone who knocks.

WORKOUT 168

With doorway stretch and one-arm lat stretch between sets, I did the following workout

CHEST AND FRONT DELTS
60-degree incline dumbbell press
45 pounds for 12 reps
30-degree incline barbell press
120 pounds 10 slow reps
pec deck
130 pounds for 12 reps
dip machine
150 pounds for 12 reps
pullover machine
140 pounds for 12 reps

TRICEPS, REAR AND SIDE DELTS
rear delt machine
90 pounds for 15 reps
pressdown
65 pounds for 12 reps
one-arm dumbbell triceps extension
30 pounds for 10 reps
one-arm dumbbell side raise
20 pounds for 12 reps
overhead triceps cable extension
50 pounds for 12 reps
pronated dumbbell side raise
12 pounds for 12 reps

ABS
hanging knee-ups
30 reps
crunches
50 reps
one-arm cable crunch
20 reps with 70 pounds
hyperextension
20 reps, followed by a one-leg up stretch

THE NATURE OF CHANGE

Infinity wears the resemblance
of my wedding to the bliss
of this world in continual flux
where nothing remains the same.
There's just no enduring self
everything changes into a metaphor
for something more
spoke the words on my lips
as I awoke in the night
dripping with insight.

WORKOUT 169

Up at the crack of dawn, I did warm-up exercises, ate breakfast, relaxed a bit then went into my *back-biceps-forearms* workout.

riding stationary bike
20 minutes

{ **leg raise**
two sets of 30 reps
crunches
two sets of 30 reps
seated twists
two sets of 30 reps

BACK

{ **front pulldown**
160 pounds for 12 reps, 175 for 10
cable crossover behind neck
40 pounds for 20 reps, 50 for 15, two arm lat stretch
between supersets

{ **low cable row**
140 pounds for 12 reps, 150 for 10
dumbbell shrug
65 pounds for 20 reps, 75 for 15

{ **close grip pulldown**
145 pounds for 12 reps, 150 for 10
reverse pec deck
55 pounds for 15 reps, 70 for 12

one-arm rowing machine
90 pounds for 12 reps, 100 for 10, one-arm lat stretch
after each set

BICEPS

one-arm dumbbell concentration curl
30 pounds for 12 reps, 35 for 10
alternate dumbbell curl
35 pounds for 12 reps, 40 for 10
preacher cable curl
80 pounds for 12 reps, 90 for 10
face down incline dumbbell curl
27 pounds for 12 reps, 30 for 10

FOREARMS

{ **barbell reverse wrist curl**
45 pounds for 10 reps, 50 for 10
barbell wrist curl
70 pounds for 15 reps, 80 for 15
gripper
two sets of 25 reps

THANKSGIVING

Today I ask
only to be what I am:
glad and free
accepting what is
there is only this
why not appreciate it?
Grateful to all who have seen fit
to sacrifice for my benefit.
Nothing else I can do

as far as I can see
I love you
because you're me.
Thanksgiving full
prayer of gratitude
and my cats yawn since
they've got nothing to do
but catch a mouse
or two.

W O R K O U T   1 7 0

I trained *abs* and *legs* today with a client in the gym at 11 A.M.:

{ **hanging knee-ups**
crunches
  both two sets of 30 reps
{ **one-arm cable crunch**
  70 pounds for 20 reps, 80 for 20 each arm
{ **hip machine**
  90 pounds for 15 reps, 100 for 15 each leg
seated twists
  100 reps

THIGHS
{ **leg extension**
  150 pounds for 12 reps, 160 for 10
{ **leg curl**
  80 pounds for 12 reps, 90 for 10 (the usual stretches in
  between)
leg press
  200 pounds for 12 reps, 220 for 10
Leg Blaster squat
  125 pounds for 12 reps, 145 for 10

CALVES
calf raises on leg press
  two sets of 15 reps, holding each rep for five seconds
  at the top
donkeys
  two sets of 15 reps, holding each rep for five seconds
  at the top
seated calf raises
  two sets of 15 reps, holding each rep for five seconds
  at the top

NO DIFFERENCE

There's no difference I'll bet
between me and this workout
since I am part of one giant set.
In reality there's no difference
between this dumbbell and me.
Yes the charm of it
is regarding that dumbbell I see
as an extension of my arm.

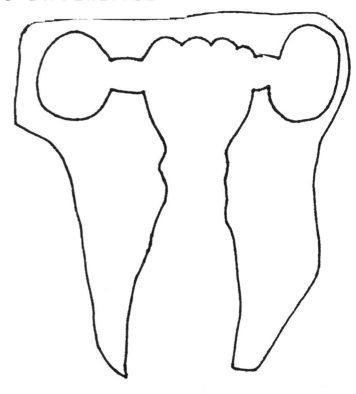

WORKOUT 171

I do a *chest-shoulder-triceps* workout today with a doorway stretch and a one-arm shoulder stretch between sets.

30-degree incline barbell press
  120 pounds for 12 reps, 140 for 10 with slow negatives
75-degree incline dumbbell press
  40 pounds for 12 reps, 45 for eight
pec deck
  115 pounds for 12 reps, 130 for 10, 145 for six
dip machine
  150 pounds for 12 reps, 160 for 10
dumbbell pullover
  70 pounds for 12 reps, 80 for 10
{ **pressdown**
  65 pounds for 12 reps, 75 for 10
rear deltoid machine
  100 pounds for 12 reps, 110 for 10
{ **one-arm dumbbell triceps extension**
  30 pounds for 10 reps, 35 for eight
one-arm side cable raise
  30 pounds for 10 reps, 30 for 10
rowing
  600 meters in three minutes

DREAM OF THE BIG KAHUNA

Awake in a dream on a tropical island beach
where a large native chief seated in peace
calls himself the big Kahuna
old but robust, alert, and wise
comes here on sunny days
and fishes for tuna.
I'm all ears as he tells me his tale
while in the distance
hear the mating call of a whale.
Man's five senses: sight, hearing, touch, taste, and smell
in Mother Earth plant seeds
eventually these become
trees, flowers, and weeds.
So inspect your behavior
weeding out unwanted tendencies
cultivating, watering, trimming, tilling the soil
to reach best bloom
everyday practice without toil
focus on your breathing
deep regular breaths ten sets of four
then make a wish
in the form of a suggestion to your animal self
just as you would train your pet
ask for your desire, your love
your animal will take it
to your angelic self above
who can fly
ascending hierarchy in the sky
delivers prayer to God Almighty.
For angels have a special relationship with animals
watching over them, animals sense this.
Your animal is like a young child
who understands everything literally
so speak to your pet with no ambiguity.
As you breathe see your being
filling with water gushing over at the top
see yourself already living your wish achieved
persist in this daily practice don't stop
this is the secret of prayer, be grateful
where three selves inhabit one body
called many names in different traditions
your animal is called lower self, id, child, subconscious instinct

you are the middle self, ego, conscious personality, the self who speaks
your angel is your higher self, guardian angel superconscious
who has a connection to your animal but not to your personality.
Do this and create what you wish,
you'll see, the Big Kahuna told me.

WORKOUT 172

Ibegan my *back-biceps-forearms* workout with the following abs and aerobics training:

{
rowing
  750 meters
leg raise
crunches
seated twist
  all: three sets of 30 reps

BACK (two-arm lat stretch between supersets)
{
front pulldown
  160 pounds for 12 reps, 170 for 10, 180 for eight
cable crossover behind neck
  40 pounds for 20 reps, 50 for 15, 60 for 10
{
low cable row
  150, 155, and 160 pounds for 10 reps
dumbbell shrug
  80 pounds for three sets of 10 reps
{
close grip pulldown
  150 pounds for 12 reps, 155 for 10
reverse pec deck
  70 pounds for 16 reps, 85 for 12
one-arm cable row
  three sets of 10 reps with 90, 100, and 110 pounds followed by a one-arm lat stretch

BICEPS AND FOREARMS
one-arm dumbbell curl
  30 pounds for 12 reps, 35 for 10, 40 for eight
face down incline dumbbell curl
  30 pounds for 12 reps, 35 for 10, 40 for eight
preacher curl
  three sets of 10 reps with 90 pounds
barbell reverse wrist curl
  two sets with 45 pounds for 12 reps
barbell wrist curl
  two sets with 80 pounds for 15 reps

BEATLES NIRVANA

Since we really are
subsets of infinity
as part of the same oneness
I am you
and you are me
and we are all together
said the walrus to the tree
to which the tree replied
So I love you because
you are me
it's impossible to
love myself
better than you
as Nirvana
said it do
before Kurt Cobain
blew out his brain.

DECEMBER 4

WORKOUT 173

I did an early morning ab-aerobic circuit, spending one minute at each station consisting of rowing, hanging knee-up, crunches, treadmill, leg raise, stationary bike, one-arm cable crunch, seated twist, two times around. It took me 20 minutes to get the effect I liked and it warmed me up for *thigh* work which I began with

hip machine
  90 pounds for 20 reps, 100 for 15
standing one-legged curl
  40 pounds for 12 reps, 45 for 10
leg extension
  150 pounds for 12 reps, 160 for 10
unlock sissy Leg Blaster squat
  100 pounds for 10 reps, 110 for 10
leg curl
  80 pounds for 12 reps, 90 for 10
leg press
  200 pounds for 12 reps, 220 for 10

  CALVES
Leg Blaster standing calf raise
  145 pounds for 12 reps, 165 for 15
calf raise on the leg press machine
  200 pounds for 15 reps, 220 for 12, holding each rep
  five seconds at the top
seated calf raise
  one set of 15 reps with 90 pounds

SWEETNESS IN LIFE

Met a man today
who uses 50 packets
of artificial sweetener a day.
I was dismayed
he had to add sweetness
to his life this way.
He wanted to know if this was too much.
All I've got to say
is it took more saccharine than this to kill laboratory rats.
We all need sweetness, we've had it all our lives
I suggest we sweeten foods in three different ways:
to sweeten cold things I use the amino acid L-glutamine
this amino increases alertness from what I've seen
for warm things the sweetest amino of all is glycine
simplest amino acid, doesn't degrade, has gh releasing properties.
The lipotropic agent inositol
is great to sweeten cold things
and is fat burning added as fuel.
These make a little artificial sweetener
go a long way feeling satisfied and full.

WORKOUT 174

This morning I did the following *chest-shoulders-triceps* training after a doorway stretch warm up:

15-degree incline barbell press
120 pounds for 15 reps, 140 for 11, 160 for nine
35-degree incline dumbbell press
55 pounds for 10 reps, 60 for nine, 65 for eight

70-degree dumbbell front press
40 pounds for 12 reps, 45 for 10, 50 for eight
pec deck
115 pounds for 15 reps, 130 for 12, 145 for 10
dip machine
150 pounds for 12 reps, 160 for 10, 170 for eight
dumbbell pullover
two sets of 10 reps with 80 pounds

DELTS AND TRICEPS
one-arm dumbbell extension
30 pounds for 12 reps, 35 for 10
one-arm dumbbell side raise
20 pounds for 12 reps, 22 for 10
pressdown
70 pounds for 12 reps, 75 for 10
rear delt machine
100 pounds for 12 reps, 110 for 10
dumbbell kickback (face down on incline bench)
22 pounds for 12 reps, 25 for 10
pronated dumbbell side raise
17 pounds for 12 reps, 20 for 10

ABS
hanging knee-ups
crunches
both three sets of 30 reps
one-arm cable crunches
30 reps with 70 pounds
seated twists
30 reps
rowed
1000 meters

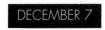

CEDAR LAKE

Late afternoon take a nap and wake up remembering a dream
of a map detailing an Indian trip in a ship sailing south
going deeper south then west finally north on rivers and into a large lake.
The full moon casts one of the eeriest shadows ever seen
as my ship sails on Cedar Lake was the theme
where I have sex making love
with a beautiful woman in my dream
as we lay beneath the moon
next to a bowl of cherries overflowing with cream.
Didn't seem like a dream
"this is real" speaks the huge beam
erected due south of my head.
"I could stay here forever" the beam said
but daylight deemed and I awake as sunlight streams
through my bedroom window and looking up I see
this instrument of my sexuality.
"Make your dream come true" it says to me
and I know my beam is far from dead
as I pole vault out of bed.

JAPAN PURE LAND

I was standing inside
the Kamakura Buddha
in Kyoto
in the land of Japan

I was walking astride
1000 golden bo dhi sat vhas
in San ju so gen do Hall
in the land of Japan

I was looking up
from the feet of the huge wooden Buddha
in Nara
in Pure Land of Japan.

I was meditating 2 days straight
sleepin on the floor
sit and contemplate
25 minutes at a time or more
get up walk around
n' sweep the floor
all my mind dust
out the door
in a temple
in Kyoto
in Pure Land Japan

I was walkin in the streets
of Osaka
ridin the bullet train
I was lookin at mount fooo jeee
in the springtime
white cherry blossoms galore
in the land of Japan

The present if just a micro-second fiction
now you see it now you don't
can't put it into diction
not even here any more
its all in my mind now
the Pure Land in Japan.

WORKOUT 175

Sex pushes and pulls
all energy
from same pool
called libido
gets used up different ways I know
workouts or sexual activity
creative driving
high octane fuel
strong solid life force
erect morning tool.
Back, biceps, forearms workout
in my gym at 11 A.M., outside it's still cool

front pulldown
 150 pounds for 12 reps, 165 for 10
cable crossover behind neck
 40 pounds for 20 reps, 50 for 15
low cable row
 145 pounds for 12 reps, 155 for 10
dumbbell shrug
 80 pounds for two sets of 15 reps
one-arm machine row
 90 pounds for 12 reps, 100 for 10, two- and one-arm
 lat stretches after all sets

 BICEPS
one-arm dumbbell concentration curl
 35 pounds two sets of 10 reps
preacher cable curl
 80 pounds for 12 reps, 90 for 10
face down incline dumbbell curl
 25 pounds for 12 reps, 30 for 10

 FOREARMS
reverse wrist curl
 40-pound fat sleeved bar two sets of 15 reps
wrist curl with Olympic bar
 80 pounds for two sets of 20 reps, shook out my
 hands

 ABS
{ **leg raise**
 crunches
 both two sets of 30 reps
seated twist
 100 reps
rowing
 750 meters in four minutes

LOADS OF PRECURSORS

Free-form amino acids muscle building blocks
peptide-bonded together form protein molecules
necessary for growth this baseline formula I use
then add two to five grams of certain aminos
to push my biochemistry in a specific direction:
L-glutamine alertness energizer brain muscle feeder
L-tyrosine mood enhancer dopamine precursor
glycine is the sweetest gh releaser of all aminos that is
L-arginine gh releaser is insulinogenic improves healing
L-leucine main branched chain promotes protein synthesis
L-tryptophan used to help me sleep tight.
In a dream I hear a new whore moan in the night
mellow tone in
drowsy delight.

REAL STATE OF THINGS

Though both body and mind appear because of cooperating causes
it does not follow that there is an ego-personality.
As the body of flesh is an aggregate of elements it is therefore, impermanent.
Neither is the mind the ego-personality.
The human mind is also an aggregate of causes and conditions.
It is in constant change.
Nothing seems to happen exactly as the ego desires.
If one is asked whether the body is constant or impermanent
he will be obliged to answer "impermanent."
If one is asked whether impermanent existence is happiness or suffering.
he will generally have to answer "suffering."
If a man believes that such impermanent a thing
so changeable and replete with suffering
is the ego-personality, it is a serious mistake.
The human mind is also impermanent and suffering.
It has nothing to be called an ego-personality.
Therefore, both body and mind, which make up an individual life
and the external world which seems to surround it
are far apart from both the conceptions of "me" and "mine."
It is simply the mind clouded over by impure desires, and impervious to wisdom
that obstinately persists of thinking of "me" and "mine."
Since both body and its surroundings are originated by cooperating causes and conditions
they are continually changing and never can come to an end.
The human mind in its never-ending change
is like the moving water of a river
or the burning flame of a candle
like an ape it is forever jumping about
not ceasing even for a moment.
Just as a picture is drawn by an artist
the human mind fills in the surroundings of its life.
All things are made up by the mind and are controlled and ruled by the mind.
Rain falls, winds blow, plants bloom, leaves mature and are blown away;
these phenomena are all interrelated with causes and conditions
and are brought about by them and disappear as causes and conditions change.
Like a net everything in this world is made up and connected by a series of ties.
Since everything in this world is caused by the concurrence and succession
of causes and conditions there can be no fundamental distinction among things.
A thing in itself does not exist so it can be said it is nonexistent.
At the same time, because of it has a relative connection with causes and conditions,
it can be said that it is not nonexistent.
A wise man seeing and hearing as such should
break away from attachment to body or mind
if he is ever to attain Enlightenment.

WORKOUT 176

Christmas vacation log cabin site
at the top of a hill
drove up here last night
stayed up until midnight I think
m,oving in Leg Blaster, dumbbells and flat/incline bench.
Awake at 8 a.m. my blender mixes a drink
with a can of Diet Rite raspberry soda quenches
my thirst mixed in a packet of whey protein
and 8 frozen strawberries
sipped slowly with 4 liver extract
2 germ oil concentrates capsule
vitamins, minerals and enzymes then
rest a bit, meditate, why I'm,
feeling fine and begin training legs at 10 a.m.

Walk down the hill 200 feet
30 degree decline
works quads and tibialis
pump up entire front of thights
jog back up
buttocks, calves, hamstrings
pump maximize

then Leg Blaster squat 3 sets of 10
100, 120, 140 pounds and then
walk back down the hill again
one-leg back stretch and
one-leg up stretch
held 15 seconds then
run back up the hill again

and do calf raise 3 sets of 15
holding 15 seconds at the top of each rep
then ran up and down the hill again
incline leg raise on the side of the hill
works lower abs great
if anything will
bunch of crunches 3 minutes or more

then did two sets of 20 leg raise
lying on the floor
then went hiking in the woods with my dog Tyler
looking for new trails to explore.

QUIET FOREST

Resting in the quiet forest I read
no blame on anyone or anything
self-cherishing attitude belongs to weaklings.
Meditating upon the kindness of problem givers
who are actually friends who bring
an opportunity to practice right thinking.

Reading put my mind at ease body at rest and
I feel relaxed all day
listening to the whisling birds and the breeze
blowing through the trees
later my blues harp wailed
a mellow tone in
the night
I felt drowsy despite
efforts to stay awake
and thought I might
partake of sleep and instead invite
myself to bed right
at that moment
I fell asleep and
had a dream that said two things:
1. Selflessness means acts done without thinking of yourself.
Its the opposite of selfishness.
2. Not only am I responsible for my own attitude
but I'm responsible for everyone else as well.
It's the entrainment thing
where my state of being
resonates through my body, my head
my entire environment.
Then saw a bright white light all around
so bright I awoke but all I found
was a dark night at 4 a.m.
so I lit a fire and went back to bed.

WORKOUT 177

I awoke to a cool morning below 30 degrees. After breakfast at a local restaurant—pass the oatmeal, please—we go window shopping, take a walk leisurely back to our cabin on the hill. Two hours later I still feel like working out, so I train my entire *upper body* with adjustable dumbbells and bench.

70-degree incline press
  35 pounds for 12 reps, 40 for 10
bent over rowing
  45 pounds for two sets of 20 reps
30-degree incline press
  two sets of 10 reps with 45 pounds
dumbbell pullover
dumbbell flys
  both two sets of ten reps with 30-pound dumbbells
  in each hand
face down incline dumbbell curls
  two sets of 10 reps with 25 pounds
dumbbell side raises
  two sets of 10 reps with 25 pounds
bent over lateral raise
  two sets with 20 pounds for 12 reps
kickbacks face down on incline bench
  two sets with 20 pounds for 12 reps

  ABS
flat bench leg raise
  two sets of 30 reps
crunches
  two sets of 50 reps
seated twists
  100 reps

then went hiking in the woods with my dog Tyler looking for new trails to explore. After dinner we left, arriving in Palm Springs just an hour later.

BLUES HARP RECORDING

Finished recording my *Train With Zane Audiotapes* today
and I was pleased if I may say they sounded more than OK.
I'd been playing harps for many days
tongue lips breathing great masses of air.
Also played Irish Tin Whistle and bell trees
Acoustics like golden angels with silver hair?
Lush reverb of my ART special effects processor
sounded very good recorded on my Yamaha four-tracker
it should with Dr. Boss rhythm section
mixed down to my Sony miniature disk recorder.
Taped holiday gift selections for friends were in order.

WORKOUT 178

Leg workout today was one giant 30-minute set combined with stretching in between:

leg extension
140 pounds for 20 reps, and one-leg back stretch
Leg Blaster squat
120 pounds for 20 reps
leg curl
80 pounds for 20 reps with one-leg up stretch
leg press
200 pounds for 20 reps
hip machine
each leg at 90 pounds for 20 reps
one-leg up stretch
standing one-leg curl
40 pounds for 20 reps
calf stretch
15 seconds
standing calf raises with Leg Blaster
150 pounds for 20 reps
calf raises on the leg press machine
180 pounds for 20 reps
seated calf raises
80 pounds for 20 reps, went for a quick drink of water

ABS
incline leg raise
50 reps
crunches
50 reps
seated twist
50 reps
stationary bike
10 minutes

THE YOGA OF SLEEP

Distorted is our sense of self while we're awake
when we fall asleep this self that is fake
dissolves into a very subtle mind
which is our real consciousness
a continuum between sleep, dreams, and being awake
it's the level of mind that remembers our dreams
living within our central nervous system landscape
behind the heart complex exists a space
a closed off chamber, a treasure box
inside a drop resides and inside this drop
the jewel of subtle consciousness abides
unrecognized but enshrined there nevertheless
sitting on a throne in a grand mansion this holiness
with no obstruction can travel anywhere
perfectly free living at home
there's nowhere it cannot roam
my heart has wings
with the golden eternal triangle inside
while all the time it sings
why hide it?

THE HAPPIEST MAN IN THE WORLD

In a dream that seemed to last all night
was a seeker of truth who with his dog and sled
over land, water, ice and snow, searched for the secret of youth
looking everywhere, there was nowhere they didn't go
crossing oceans, dense jungles, dark forested mountains filled with strife
until finally the seeker met a wise old man living with his wife
at the base of an azure blue mountain running through the desert.
Begging the old man for the secret of eternal life
the old man replied, "Use this map to find the cocoon of immortality
which lies in a deep cavern beneath the sea."
Reaching the destination indicated by the map
the seeker dove to the bottom of the sea and searching finds
the passage to this underworld. Crawling through tunnels thinking it's a trap
he eventually enters a cavern where a cocoon hangs from the branch of a tree.
As he touches the cocoon it splits in two and out flies a massive
Golden Monarch Butterfly whose giant wing brushes against the side of his head
plunging him into a deep sleep. Dreaming he hears
"You must find the happiest man in the world now you see
buy his shirt, put it on and wear it home. You'll learn the secret of immortality
and all you meet will be made younger instantly."
Then the Golden Butterfly guided the seeker from the depths
of the cave up from the waters of the deep and he awakens on the beach.
After following the butterfly for a long time over all kinds of terrain
the seeker realizes he is the Golden Butterfly and begins to fly
and comes to a gate in the desert at the foot of a huge snow-capped peak
enclosing an estate hidden by dense foliage as laughter reverberates the sky
from inside the seeker opens the gate to find an old man laughing hysterically.
"I have never heard laughter such as this before. You must be the happiest man
in the world. I wish to buy your shirt and will pay whatever you ask or even more.
Please give me the shirt off your back so I can wear it for all to see" said the seeker.
"If you had only taken the trouble to look" said the happiest man "you would see
that I do not possess a shirt. I am only the humble caretaker of this estate."
"What do I do now?" asked the seeker. The happiest man replied,
"You will now be cured. Striving for something unattainable provides the exercise
to achieve that which is needed: as a man gathers all his strength to jump
across a stream as if it were far wider than it is. He gets across the stream, wise.
Haven't you ever seen any Jackie Chan movies?" When the happiest man
who had been talking with his back to the seeker turned around
the seeker saw he was the same wise old man who he had come to seek advice
from many years before. "But why did you not tell me all this years ago
when I first came to see you?" the restless seeker asked, he didn't know.
"Because you were not ready then to understand. You needed certain experiences
and they had to be given to you in a manner that would ensure that you
go through them."
Waking up, I wrote out the dream and came to my senses.

FULL CIRCLE

Looking back, three states of being need cultivation in fact:
calm
appreciation
love
be calm at all times
deep relaxation follows exercise
nurture the intellect and creative spirit
through music writing art reading heart math
meditate regularly on sound
stay on the path both feet on the ground
relaxed calm will abound.
Set aside time each day to appreciate someone and something special.
In my mind each person's superimposed on a heart with wings
golden triangle in a red hearted field flies out, sends and brings
things I need you could use too. Here's what to do:
First thank your body for supporting you with a place to live.
This is your being.
Thank your body for not always being in the place where you want to be
otherwise there would be no place to go.
This is your goal.
Thank your body for being your energy vehicle to get there.
This is your motivation.
Thank your body for being a spacious home for your three selves:
    physical animal id of instincts
    logical rational ego personality being in the world self that acts and speaks
    angelic higher spiritual self, bodhimind, subtle vehicle
Enlightened Self Golden Eternal Butterfly Heart Wings
three deeds of thought, speech, and action
pack the Golden Triangle vertices with things
needed at all times to
have the right attitude
with direction straight on course
you will surely succeed as appreciation becomes love's powerful force.

YEAR END

Now another year is vanishing into the past
and I'm back to where I began my quest.
Have I reached my goal? If the path is the goal
then the quest is what teaches best
that only the end in itself has meaning.
Now I see it's not the assumption of what the end might be.
Whatever it is, I'm getting ready to do it all over again.
Let the wheel continue to spin
amen until the end when even then
I will win.

WINTER CACTUS GROWING

Cactus are growing in the cold moonlight
but need trimming, I see
where once there was one
now there are three.
Cactus are growing in the void
filling it with something to be.
Cactus of morning came and left
and it was afternoon all over again.
Cactus are growing after the afternoon
and into the fright full night.
Cactus are a growing
moon light silhouette on the ground
My body is a growing
shadow on the moon
cast by reflecting earth light
body cactus silhouette
on moon and ground all around.

Then thoughts about training
think layoffs are ok but already
planning to start up again
and when I do I will train a day
rest a day or two, an easy life
and more fun to get enough rest
ease is essential to grow your best and
heal injuries.

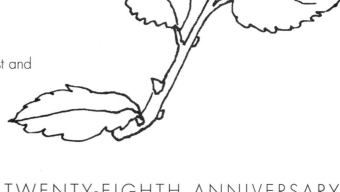

TWENTY-EIGHTH ANNIVERSARY

Reflecting inside
my fire's exploding
the sparks sprinkle
a fresh log roaring
warms the Palm Springs winter.
Misty morning clouds alight
abated rains reveal
majestic snowy peaks delight.
Abyss

a bliss
rainy realm
snow before Christmas.
New rosebuds
in the frosty chill of early morning
pick one
then two
love you.

MESSAGE NOT MEDIUM

Christ or Buddha
what's it to ya
not the medium
but the message
don't let it fool ya
it's not a matter
of who you believe
but what's being said.
I learned that all the great
spiritual teachings led
to the same end:
be nice practice
empathy and kindness
nothing to lose
by putting yourself
in another's shoes.

CHRISTMAS EVE

Bitter sweet cold morning
calls a songbird's shrill message
as mists rise from pools of still waters
white spiral mountain cathedrals glisten in the sun.
Precipitous white powder on immense vaulted masses
radiating luxurious splendor in such cold morning sunlight
I could see my breath and ponder my quest for meaning.
Is it just more grist for the mill?
But not going to bed
we get a thrill by opening gifts instead.
Find a fountain pen and ink for Christine
and a chromatic harmonica in the key of F for me.
We write and play immediately.

CHRISTMAS

With Christmas comes the spirit of giving
taught me by Cherry, my first tree.
We were children growing up at 11 Franklin Street
in my backyard.
You were many things to me:
a chin up bar
place to hang out in and eat
sweet summer fruit always free
wood carvings from a fallen branch
a home for wildlife
shelter from the sun
climbing high in my hiding place was fun
on moonless nights.
Caterpillars eventually killed my tree.
Sometimes I wonder
if her spirit flew away
on the wings of
10,000 butterflies.

THE DAY AFTER CHRISTMAS

Awake with the sunlight of a new morning
that casts long menacing shadows
in the mountains rocky crags called
the Witch of Tahquitz according to Indian legend
cast a spell, kind of chasm sarcasm feeling here still
the biggest sale day of the year will be today
so Christine goes shopping early
for next year's Christmas frill.
My dog Tyler paces a perimeter inspection
for anything needing barking protection.
Warming up to 43 degrees in the shade
training not too much I'm afraid.
Winter layoff said I'd rest today
but walked an 18-minute
mile on my treadmill anyway.

COLD MORNING IMAGERY

A bleak cloudy dawn
unaware of its 40 degrees
saw me take out the garbage
in her desert dream.
With morning still asleep
waiting for inspiration
eyes watching ideas
behind closed eyelids
energy flows freely
to the sight of sound
10 to 13 hertz beat frequency tape.
Images abound dreaming in trance
suddenly I feel awake
wandering in woods
where weeds cover the fat of the land
seeking a path grown over
but well worn and deep
many years of travel reveal
footprints in a deserted field.
Still searching, wake up . . .
it seemed so real
as words flash to mind:
"Since you travel
these woods all the time
the path you seek
will not be hard to find."

ELICITING THE RELAXATION RESPONSE IN LIEU OF SLEEP

My early morning spiritual practice
goes from active to passive
cause to effect hierarchy
topping the list is:

1. Spontaneous writing
   enhance my creative ability
   jot first thoughts freely.

2. Prayer, positive id suggestion
   ask to receive.

3. Mantra repetition
   sometimes quite a while.

4. Traditional meditation
   enlightenment smile.

5. Light and sound entrainment
   more than mere entertainment.

6. Dichotic and beat frequency
   audio tapes free relaxation ability.

7. Harmonica straight and cross harp
   diatonic and chromatic
   green bullet mike
   amped up special effects
   reverbs my psyche.

8. Hearing sounds tones and chords
   with my whole body
   lying on my sound table affords
   muscle bone resonation
   deepest relaxation I've known.

9. Guiding the body's electrical
   microcurrent with copper biocircuit
   I think there's more
   than a placebo effect to it.

10. Cranial electrical stimulation relieving pain
    with probes in earlobes
    throbs diffuse three dimensionally.

These top 10
restore my energy
revitalize my spirit
enhance creativity.

With winter layoff almost complete
I play harp singin' blues
composing new songs
all with four beats:

DEATH FEARIN' BLUES

Death fearin' blues
in everything I do
this fact of dyin'
gotta admit it's true.
In everything I do.

Everybody you see
happenin to them too
I'happen to you n' me.
In ev it a bil ity.
Will happen to you n' me.

Fear of death
that's what you get
that's what you got
death fearin' blues
it's not so hot.

Death fearin blues
feel pain all the time.
Death fearin blues
can't get em outta my mind.
Working over time.

LOSE DEATH FEARIN' BLUES

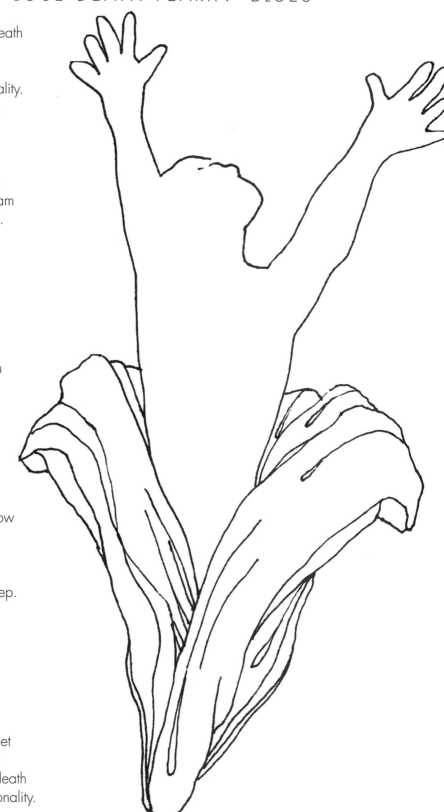

Conquer fear of death
be all you can be
transform yourself
high self is personality.
Be all you can be.

At time of death
like in a dream
blow yr last breath
bending angel beam
jus like in a dream.

Unconscious mind
down in the deep
death's just like
fallin asleep
mind in the deep.

Wake up in dream
new real ality.
Ex per ee ence
your new body
new real ality.

Know you know how
to fall fast asleep.
Just let go
trust real deep.
Go deep deep deep.

Make the most
of what you got
build dream body
fear not a lot
really all ya got.

That's what you'll get
birth of new reality.
Transcend fear of death
go beyond impersonality.

Birth to new reality.

Yes it's true
same for me n you
build spiritual self
new year, new you.
End death fearin blues.

PLANETARY CONSCIOUSNESS

As one tiny cell
in the body of earth
just as my fingers
are part of me
living breathing free
earth dirt collects under my nails
this ego is due for sure
manicure.
Gathering experience
growing mature
todding on, seeking how to improve
using life situations
as motivation to move me
toward the goal on this path
widens into a road at last
of unknown destination.

Now the trees
have lost their leaves
but growth is still to be found
as roots drink life fluid
a vast network expands
deep underground.
Just as the roots
create the future tree
in this present life abounds
the possibility
of your next body.

Winter's peering right around
the corner.

AUTUMN WORKOUT SUMMARY

DATE	MY WORKOUT	YOUR WORKOUT
September 22	back, biceps, forearms, abs, aerobics	
September 23	thighs, calves, abs	
September 24	chest, shoulders, triceps, abs, aerobics	
September 25	posing	
September 26	posing	
September 28	competition	
October 1	back, biceps, forearms, abs	
October 2	thighs, calves, abs	
October 4	chest, shoulders, triceps, abs	
October 6	back, biceps, forearms, abs, aerobics	
October 7	aerobics, thighs, calves, abs	
October 8	chest, shoulders, triceps, abs	
October 10	chest, back, abs	
October 12	thighs, calves, abs	
October 14	delts, arms, abs	
October 16	back, biceps, forearms, thighs, calves	
October 18	chest, shoulders, triceps, abs	
October 21	back, biceps, forearms, thighs, calves, abs	
October 23	chest, shoulders, triceps, abs	
October 26	thighs, calves	
October 28	chest, shoulders, triceps, abs	
October 30	back, biceps, forearms, abs	
November 1	thighs, calves, abs	
November 4	curl, bench press, deadlift	
November 7	upper body	
November 8	thighs, calves, abs	
November 10	full body	
November 13	full body	
November 15	aerobics, full body	

November 17	abs
November 18	upper body
November 20	back, biceps, forearms, abs
November 22	abs, thighs, calves
November 24	chest, shoulders, triceps, abs
November 26	aerobics, back, biceps, forearms, abs
November 28	abs, thighs, calves
November 30	chest, shoulders, triceps, aerobics
December 2	back, biceps, forearms
December 4	ab-aerobics, thighs, calves
December 6	chest, shoulders, triceps, abs, aerobics
December 9	back, biceps, forearms, abs
December 12	thighs, calves, abs
December 14	upper body
December 16	thighs, calves, abs, aerobics
December 26	aerobics

EXCERCISES

THIGHS

Leg Extension

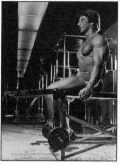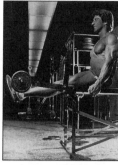

Sit on leg extension machine, placing ankles behind the bottom rollers, push up against the rollers so that your legs are extended as you exhale, slowly allow your legs to return to starting position, inhaling.

Leg Curl

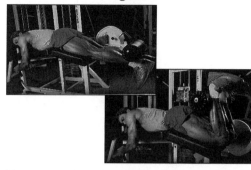

Lie on your stomach with legs fully extended and knees slightly over the end of the table pad. With your heels under the roller pad and holding the handles on the sides, slowly curl your heels up to your rear inhaling, then slowly lower your heels back to the extended position as you exhale.

Leg Press

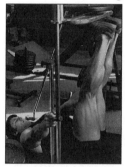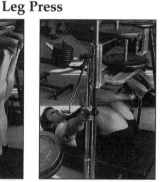

With the angle of the machine properly adjusted, sit in the leg press machine with your feet on the pushing plate, press the plate up and release the restraining handles; bend your knees to lower the weight plate as you inhale, then slowly press your legs to the fully extended position, exhaling.

Leg Blaster Squat

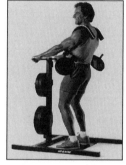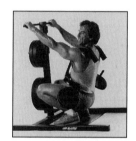

With the weights draped across your shoulders and holding onto the handle bars, slowly lower into a squat with your head and chest up, inhaling, then return to the upright position as you exhale.

Barbell Squat

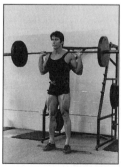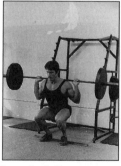

Step into the squat rack to place a barbell across your shoulders. While gripping the bar wider than your shoulders, slowly lower into a squat inhaling; when returning to an upright position, keep your head and chest up as you exhale.

Front Squat

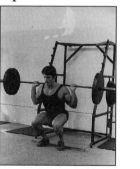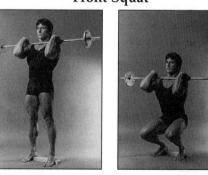

While standing, grasp the barbell with your hands at about shoulder width and hold it across your upper chest; with your upper body erect, slowly lower yourself to a squat, inhaling, then slowly push yourself to standing erect as you exhale.

Hip Machine

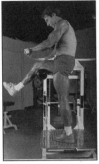 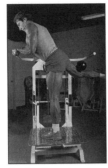

While standing on one leg and with the other leg on top of the roller pad, inhaling, slowly swing the roller from in front of you (with your knee pointing straight ahead) to fully behind you as you exhale.

Sissy Squat

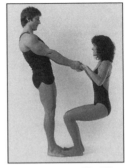

Facing a partner, toe-to-toe and holding hands, inhaling, slowly bend your knees to a full squat position while keeping your upper body erect, then return to standing position as you exhale.

Lunges

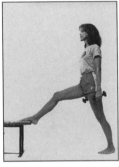 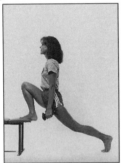

While standing erect and holding dumbbells or barbell, inhaling, take one long step forward and lower your body until your rear knee touches the floor. Shift your weight backward to return to upright position as you exhale.

One-Legged Curl

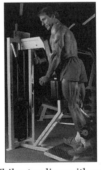 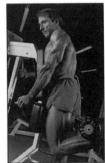

While standing with your heels under the roller pad and holding onto the handles, slowly curl the heel of one leg up towards your rear as you inhale, then slowly lower the leg back to the extended position, exhaling.

One-Leg Top Extension

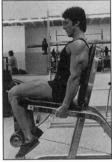 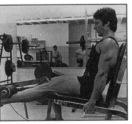

While sitting on the leg extension machine with your knees at the end of the seat and ankles under the bottom roller, slowly push up against the roller with one leg until your leg is completely extended, inhaling, then return your leg to a half way down position as you exhale.

Hack Squat

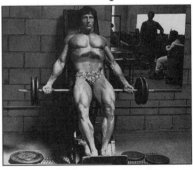

Lying back into the hack squat machine with your shoulders under the pads, press up until your legs are fully extended, exhaling, then bend your knees and lower your body into a squat as you inhale, return to upright position by straightening your legs.

Hack Squat with Dumbbells

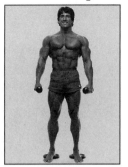 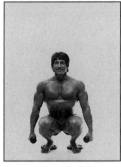

With heels on a 2-by-4 block grasp a dumbbell in each hand, inhale as you squat slowly as low as possible, and exhale as you return to start position.

Stiff-Legged Deadlift

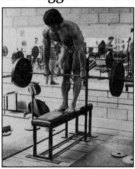

Grasping a barbell with a shoulder-width grip, inhale as you bend forward at the waist, keeping knees locked. Go as low as you can and exhale as you return to the starting position.

Quarter Squat

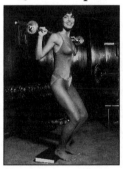

Same as regular squat except squat only one quarter of the way down inhaling and exhale as you return to starting position.

CALVES

Standing Calf Raise

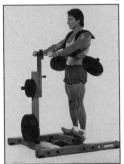 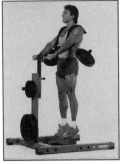

Step into a standing calf raise machine, positioning your toes on the block with heels extended off the edge, keeping knees slightly bent, raise up on your toes, hold for up to five seconds, then slowly lower heels toward floor as far as they will go.

Donkey Calf Raise

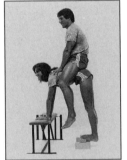 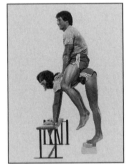

Have a training partner sit on your lower back while you are holding on to a support and standing on the edge of a narrow platform with your heels extended off the edge, slowly raise up on your toes, holding at the top up to five seconds, then lower heels toward the floor as far as they will go.

One-Legged Calf Raise

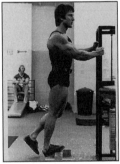 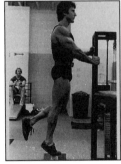

Same as standing calf raise, but with only one foot on the block while the other is slightly raised behind you.

Seated Calf Raise

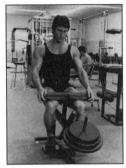 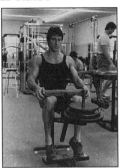

Sitting on calf machine with the balls of your feet on the foot plate, slowly raise your heels up as high as they will go, hold for up to five seconds, then lower your heels until they are as low as they can go.

Leg Press Calf Raise

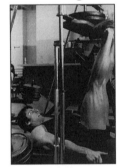 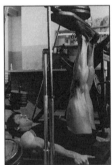

Assume leg press position with heels hanging off edge of platform, push toes up as high as possible, hold up to five seconds, then lower heels, stretching as low as you can go.

Calf Raise Face Down
on Hack Machine

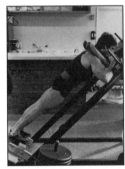 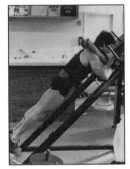

Lying face down in the hack machine with your heels extended over the bottom inclined platform, slowly raise and lower your heels while keeping your body straight.

BACK

Front Pulldown

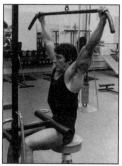 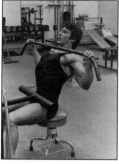

Sitting in pulldown machine with your legs under the brace, slowly pull down the bar until it reaches your chest as you inhale, then return slowly the bar to the starting position as you exhale.

Low Cable Row

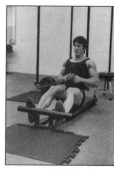

While sitting upright on a low cable pulley machine with knees slightly bent and with your feet braced at the foot plate, grasp the cable handles and pull them to your ribcage as you exhale, then return slowly to the starting position as you inhale.

Dumbbell Shrug

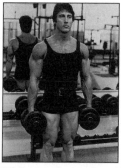 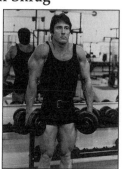

While standing erect and holding a dumbbell in each hand with your arms at your sides, slowly raise your shoulders as high as they will go, then lower shoulders as low as they will go.

One-Arm Dumbbell Row

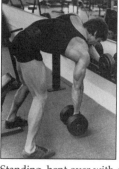 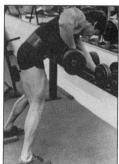

Standing bent over with one hand bracing your body and knees bent, with other hand pull up a dumbbell to side of chest inhaling and lower dumbbell one inch from the floor as you exhale.

One-Arm Cable Row

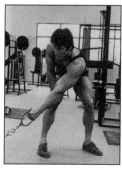 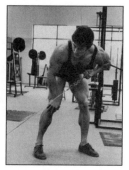

Bent over with one hand braced on your knee, pull the low cable toward your chest touching side of pec as you inhale, then slowly return it to the starting position, stretching way out as you exhale.

Cable Crossover Behind Neck

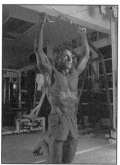 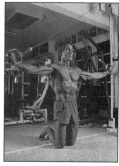

Grasp a cable handle overhead with each hand, exhaling as you lower each hand to the side, slowly returning handles to overhead as you inhale.

Close Grip Pulldown

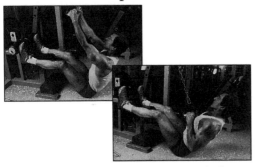

Grab the lat pulley handles while sitting on the floor in front of the lat machine with your heels elevated on the seat. Inhale as you pull the handles to your solar plexis, keeping your elbows in, shoulders back and chest pulled up. Exhale as you slowly return the handles to the start position, stretching as far as you can in this position.

Pulldown Behind Neck

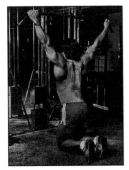 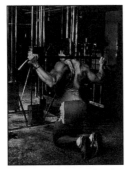

Sitting in pulldown machine with your legs under the brace, slowly pull down the bar behind your neck until it reaches your shoulders as you inhale, then return the bar to the starting position exhaling.

T-Bar Row (Leverage Row)

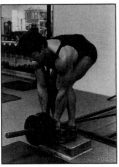 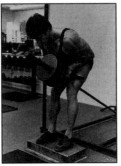

Bent forward at waist and standing over the T-bar machine, pull the T-bar up to your chest inhaling, then lower to the starting position as you exhale, all the while keeping your knees slightly bent.

Barbell Row

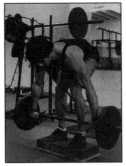 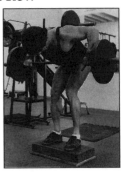

Bending forward at the waist with a barbell straight down in front, slowly lift the barbell up as you inhale until it reaches your chest, then slowly lower it to the starting position, exhaling.

One-Arm Rowing Machine

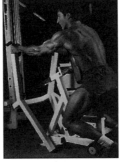 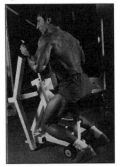

Sitting sideways in a rowing machine with waist against support, use one hand to pull handle into your waist as you inhale, then return to start position exhaling.

Deadlift

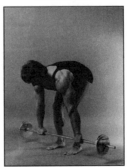

Squat down with upper body straight to grasp the barbell at your feet, then slowly raise your body by straightening your knees and holding the barbell with your arms straight.

Top Deadlift

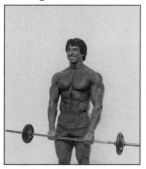

Using a power rack grasp bar slightly above knees and inhale as you pull bar up by straightening legs and upper body. Return to start as you exhale.

Hyperextension

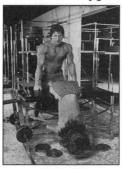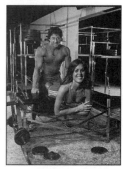

Lying bent over hyperextension machine with legs under the roller pad and head near the ground, slowly raise your upper torso so that it is parallel to the ground as you inhale, then return to starting position, exhaling.

Front Chin

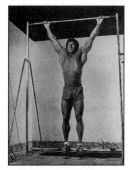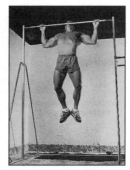

Gripping bar with your hands fully extended over your head, pull your chin up to the bar, inhaling, then slowly lower your body as you exhale.

Good Morning Exercise

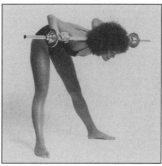

Standing erect with barbell across your shoulders, bend at your hips as you exhale until your upper body is parallel to the floor, then return to upright position, inhaling.

CHEST

Dumbbell Fly

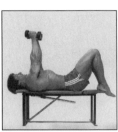
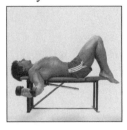

Lying on your back on a bench with a dumbbell in each hand with arms extended overhead with elbows slightly bent, lower the dumbbells out to your sides to shoulder level, inhaling, then slowly return to overhead position as you exhale.

Incline Barbell Press

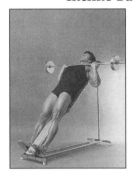
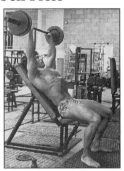

Lying back down on an inclined bench, grasp a barbell over your chest and press them overhead until your arms are extended with elbows slightly unlocked as you exhale, then return the barbell to your chest, inhaling.

Incline Dumbbell Press

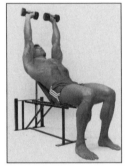
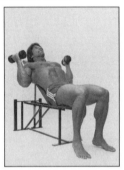

Same as incline barbell press but with a dumbbell in each hand instead of a barbell.

Incline Press on Smith Machine

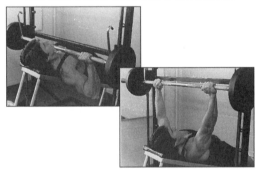

Same as incline barbell press but using a Smith Machine.

Pec Deck

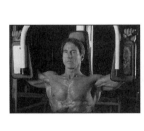
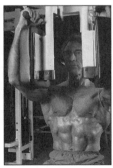

Sitting upright in a pec deck machine with arms bent at the elbow and out to each side, grip the pads on each side of your body and slowly move them to a position in front of you exhaling, then return to start as you inhale.

Dumbbell Pullover

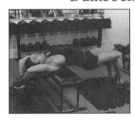
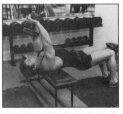

Lying across a flat bench, hold a dumbbell with both hands with elbows slightly bent, slowly lower the dumbbell behind your head keeping elbows bent at same angle as you inhale. Lower your arms below level of bench, then return to start as you exhale.

Dip Machine

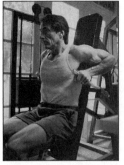 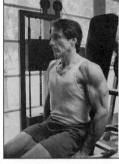

Sitting in dip machine, grip handles on each side, press down from chest high as you exhale, then slowly return to start, inhaling.

Cable Crossover

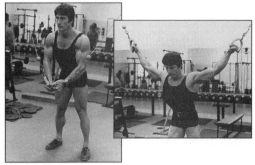

Grasp cable pulley handles in each hand above the head while standing erect, pull the handles down crossing your wrists in front of your body as you exhale, then return to starting position, and inhale.

Decline Dumbbell Press

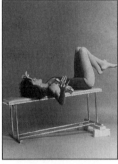 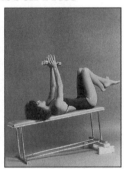

Lying on tilted bench with your head at the lowest end, press the dumbbells from your chest directly above you as you exhale, then slowly lower the dumbbells to your chest, inhaling.

Decline Dumbbell Fly

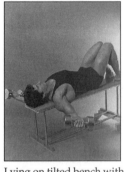 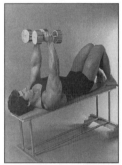

Lying on tilted bench with your head at the lowest end and a dumbbell in each hand with arms extended overhead with elbows slightly bent, move the dumbbells out to your sides to shoulder level, as you inhale, then slowly return to overhead position exhaling.

Incline Dumbbell Fly

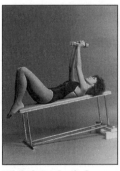 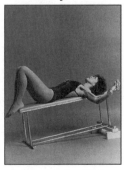

While lying back down on an incline bench with your feet flat on the floor, grasp two dumbbells overhead with arms slightly bent at the elbows, move the dumbbells out to your sides as low as they will go as you inhale, then return to the overhead position exhaling.

Bench Press

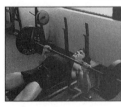 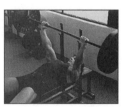

Lying back down on a bench, grasp a barbell from the rack above you with a shoulder width grip, hold the barbell above you and slowly lower it to your chest inhaling, then press back up just short of lockout.

Parallel Dip

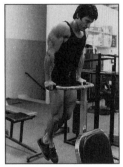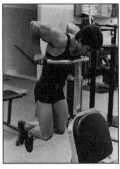

Standing erect, grasp the dip bars to support yourself with arms fully extended and knees bent, slowly lower yourself as far as possible inhaling, then slowly press your body up to the starting position as you exhale.

Stiff-Arm Pulldown

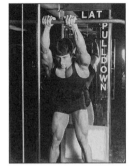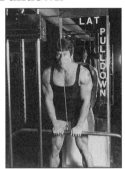

Standing upright, grasp pulldown bar with arms fully extended and pull it down in front of you with slightly bent elbows as you exhale, then raise to the overhead position again, inhaling.

SHOULDERS

Seated Dumbbell Front Press

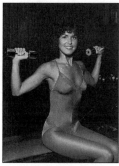 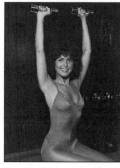

Sitting on the end of a bench with feet on the floor, hold two dumbbells next to shoulders, with back straight slowly press dumbbells straight overhead exhaling, then lower to shoulder level as you inhale.

70-Degree Incline Dumbbell Press

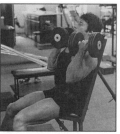 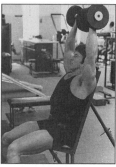

Same as seated dumbbell front press, but done on a bench angled at 70 degrees.

Dumbbell Rear Deltoid Raises

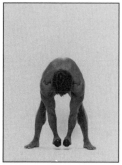 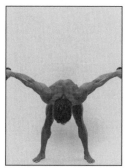

Sitting on end of a bench with feet on the floor (or stand bending forward at waist), bend down to grasp a dumbbell in each hand, slowly raise them out to the side until the extended arms are parallel to the floor with arms slightly bent at elbows exhaling, then slowly lower them to the floor as you inhale.

Rear Delt Machine
(Reverse Pec Deck)

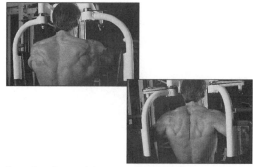

Stepping forward into pec deck machine, with your arms bent at the elbows and parallel to the floor, place the back of your triceps against pads, and press the pads as far back as you can go exhaling, then return your arms to the front as you inhale.

One-Arm Side Cable Raise

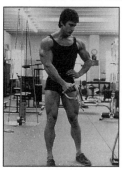 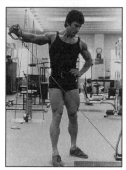

While standing sideways, grasp a low pulley handle with an opposite hand, pull across your body until your arm is fully extended parallel to the floor exhaling, then return to the start as you inhale.

One-Arm Side Dumbbell Raise

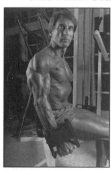 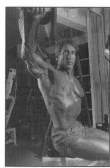

With dumbbell in one hand (elbow slightly bent) while holding on to a vertical pole with the other, raise and lower the dumbbell slowly with fully extended arm straight down to straight out to the side.

Pronated Side Dumbbell Raise

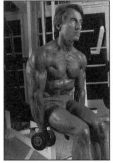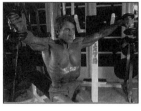

From a sitting position, hold a dumbbell pronated in each hand with thumbs pointing straight down, slowly raise your fully-extended arms out to the sides until they are parallel with the floor inhaling, then slowly lower them as you exhale.

Two-Arm Side Dumbbell Raise

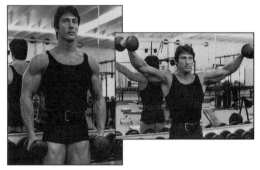

Standing with a dumbbell in each hand and arms at your sides, slowly raise the dumbbells to the side until they are at ear level inhaling, then slowly lower them to the start as you exhale.

Dumbbell Upright Rowing

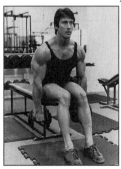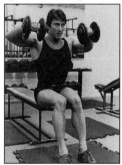

While sitting on the edge of a bench with each hand on a dumbbell, pull the dumbbells straight up the front of your body, touch your chin or top of chest as you inhale, exhaling as you lower to start.

Bent-Over Rear Delt Cable Raise

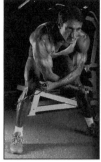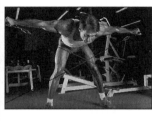

While bending over at the hips, grasp low pulley handles in opposite hands (with arms bent at the elbows), slowly raise the handles out to your sides as high as you can go with arms extended exhaling, then slowly return the handles to the starting position inhaling.

Barbell Press Behind the Neck

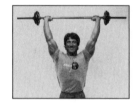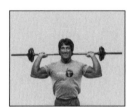

Sitting on a bench, grasp the barbell and bring it to shoulder level behind your neck, keeping the elbows to the outside, slowly press the bar up until your arms are fully extended overhead as you exhale, then return as you inhale.

Machine Press

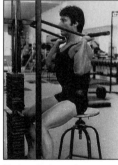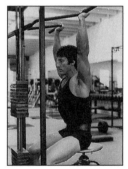

Sitting facing a front press machine, grasp the bar, then slowly press the bar until your arms are extended overhead as you exhale, then return it to starting position as you inhale.

One Dumbbell Front Raise

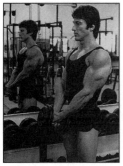 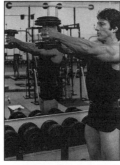

Standing while grasping one dumbbell with both hands in front, slowly raise the dumbbell until your arms are fully extended straight out in front inhaling, then lower to the starting position as you exhale.

Two-Dumbbell Front Raise

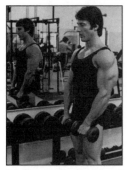 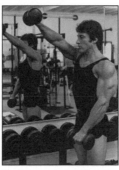

While standing with a dumbbell in each hand, raise one dumbbell from thigh level to straight out in front, alternating the raise with each arm. Exhale as you raise the dumbbell, inhale as it is lowered.

Rear Delt Face Down Incline Dumbbell Raise

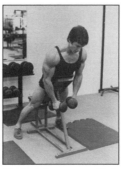 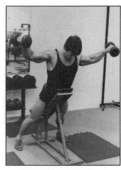

Lie face down on a 45-degree inclined bench, holding a dumbbell in eachhand. Inhale as you raise the dumbbells out to each side, twisting the wrists outward as you raise them. The dumbbells should be slightly forward. Exhale as you slowly lower the dumbbells to the starting position.

Barbell Clean and Press Overhead

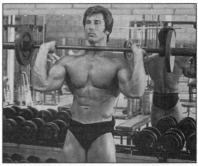

From a standing position and holding a barbell with both hands straight down in front, exhale and slowly raise the barbell up to a rest position at chin level and inhale with arms fully bent at the elbows, exhale as you press the barbell straight overhead, then inhale as you return to the starting position.

BICEPS

Barbell Curl

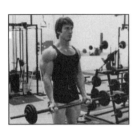 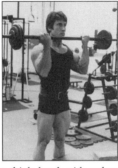

Standing, holding barbell at thigh level with palms facing away from you, curl it up to your chin with upper arm stationary as possible, inhaling. Lower slowly to start as you exhale.

One-Arm Dumbbell Concentration Curl

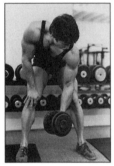 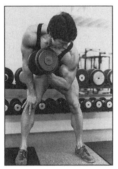

Bent over with one hand holding a dumbbell which is resting on the floor and the other resting on a knee, exhale as you raise the dumbbell up to your face by only moving your forearm and bending at the elbow, then inhale as you slowly lower the dumbbell to the floor.

Incline Dumbbell Curl

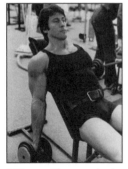 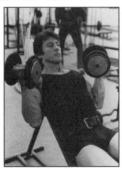

Sitting with your back resting against an inclined bench while holding a dumbbell in each hand (arms straight down), exhale as you slowly curl the dumbbells to shoulder level by bending at the elbows (pointed straight down), then inhaling, slowly return the dumbbells towards the floor with arms fully extended.

Face Down Incline Dumbbell Curl

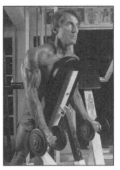 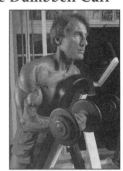

Lying face down on an inclined bench with a dumbbell in each hand (underhand grip), exhale as you raise the dumbbells from straight down in front to your chest by bending at the elbows, then inhale as you slowly lower them back to the start.

Preacher Cable Curl

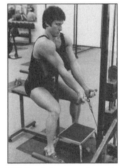 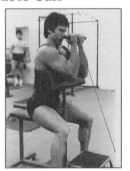

While sitting on the edge of a bench, grasp a low pulley handle with both hands and arms straight out in front, exhale as you pull the handle up to your face by bending at the elbows, then inhaling, slowly return to straight out in front.

Alternate Dumbbell Curl

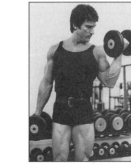 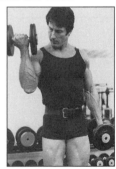

Standing while holding a dumbbell in each hand (arms straight down), exhale as you slowly curl one dumbbell from thigh to shoulder level by bending at the elbow, then inhaling slowly return to the starting position, and repeat with the other arm.

Seated One-Arm Dumbbell Curl

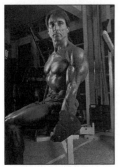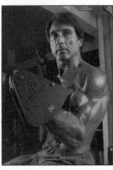

Sitting on a bench with a dumbbell in one hand and the other hand resting on your knee, curl the dumbbell up to the side of your head by bending at the elbow as you inhale, then return to start, exhaling.

Barbell Preacher Curl

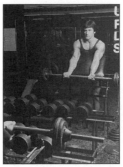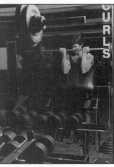

Both elbows on a preacher bench and holding a barbell with an underhanded grip, exhale as you slowly curl the barbell up towards your face until your arms are flexed, then inhale as you return your arms to the fully extended position.

TRICEPS

Pressdown

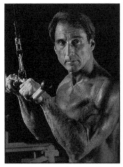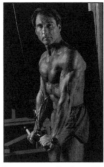

Standing in front of a high pulley, grasp the handle with both hands at chest level and elbows bent, exhale as you slowly press down on the handle until your arms are fully extended in front of you, then inhale as you slowly return the handle to chest level.

One-Arm Dumbbell Extension

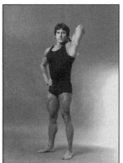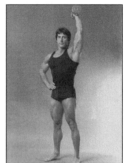

While sitting on the end of a bench, hold a dumbbell overhead with your arm fully extended , inhale as you slowly lower it behind your head as far back as it will go, then exhale as you return the dumbbell directly overhead.

Close Grip Bench Press

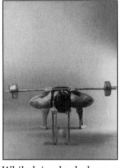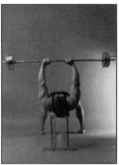

While lying back down on a bench (feet on the floor) and holding a barbell with a narrow grip on your chest exhale as you, slowly press the barbell straight above you, then inhale as you slowly return the bar to your chest.

Cable Extension

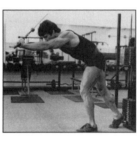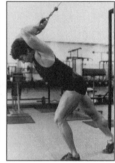

Bending forward at the waist, grasp a thick rope or curved bar attached to an overhead pulley, and as you exhale, straighten your arms then return to start, inhaling.

Dumbbell Kickbacks

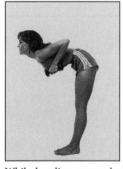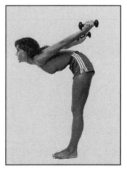

While bending over a bench and supporting yourself with one hand and a knee on the bench, hold a dumbbell in the other hand such that your elbow is bent and the upper arm is against your body, exhale as you extend your forearm to the rear until it is fully extended and above your back, then inhale as you return to the start.

EZ Bar Overhead Extension

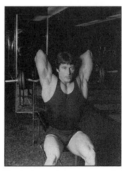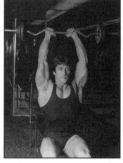

Seated, grasp a curved bar behind your neck, and keeping elbows close to your head, extend the bar overhead as you exhale. Return slowly to start, inhaling.

Lying Triceps Extension

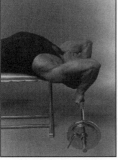 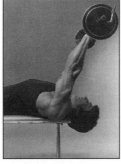

Hold a dumbbell overhead with both hands (elbows bent) while lying back down on a bench, keeping your upper arms and elbows stationary inhale as you bend the dumbbell behind your head as far as it will go, then exhale as you return to starting position.

One-Arm Cable Kickback

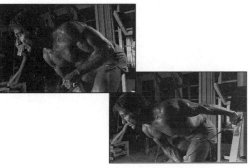

In a standing position, bend over and brace yourself with one hand on a knee and the other hand grasping a low pulley (arm bent), exhale as you pull the handle directly in back of you with your arm fully extended and parallel to the floor, then inhale as you return to the start.

Reverse Triceps Dips

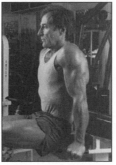 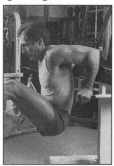

With hands holding parallel bars or the edge of a bench, your arms completely bent, and legs straight out in front of you, exhale as you push yourself up, tensing triceps, inhale as you slowly descend into start position.

One-Dumbbell Triceps Extension (with Two Arms)

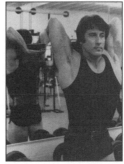 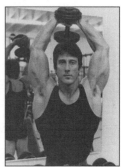

Hold a dumbbell overhead with both hands (elbows bent) while sitting on a bench, keeping your upper arms and elbows stationary inhale as you lower the dumbbell behind your head as far as it will go, then exhale as you return to starting position.

FOREARMS

Barbell Reverse Curl

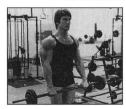
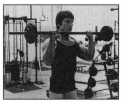

While standing and holding a barbell straight down in front of you with an overhand grip, exhale as you raise the barbell to your chin by bending your elbows, then inhale as you return to start.

Barbell Wrist Curl

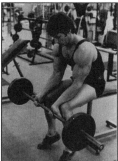
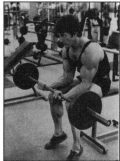

Sitting on the end of a bench with forearms resting on your legs, hold a barbell with an underhand grip, exhale as you slowly raise and inhale as you lower your hands by bending at the wrists.

Hand Grippers

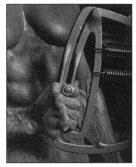

Squeeze and release the grippers.

EZ Bar Reverse Grip Preacher Curl

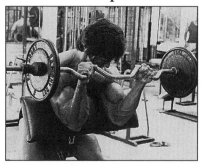

With upper arms on a preacher bench and holding an EZ bar with an overhand grip, exhale as you raise the barbell to your chin by bending your elbows, then inhale as you return to start.

Barbell Reserve Wrist Curl

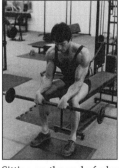
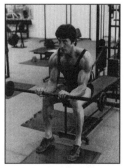

Sitting on the end of a bench with forearms resting on your legs, hold a barbell with an overhand grip exhale as you, slowly raise and inhale as you lower your hands by bending at the wrists.

ABS

Hanging Knee-Up

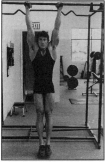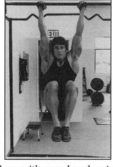

Hanging from a chinning bar with overhand grip, slowly bend your knees as you exhale and lift your legs as high as possible, then return to starting position inhaling.

Crunch

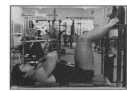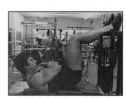

Lying on your back with legs in the air, exhale as you slowly raise your head and hips simultaneously off the floor as high as they will go. Hold for two seconds, then slowly lower your head and hips to the floor as you inhale.

Seated Twist

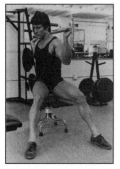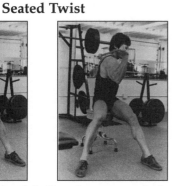

While sitting on a bench, hold a pole across your back, and slowly turn your upper body as far as it will go to the left, then to the right.

One-Arm Cable Crunch

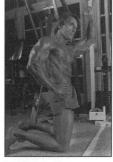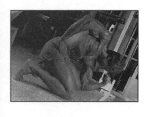

While kneeling, grasp a high pulley cable handle with one hand above your head (the other hand on your hip), exhale as you slowly bend your upper body until your elbow touches the floor, then inhale as you return to start.

Leg Raise

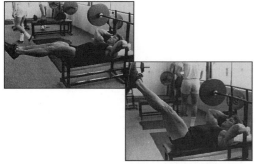

Lying back down on a bench and grasping the sides, exhale as you raise and inhale as you lower both legs from a fully extended position to a 45-degree angle.

Partial Situp

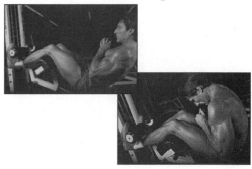

Lying on your back with legs bent at a 45-degree angle and arms on your chest, exhale as you curl your upper body until your forearms touch your thighs, then exhale as you slowly lower to the starting position.

Pulley Knee-In

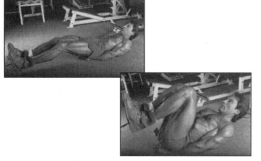

Lying on your back, legs together and straight out in front, with low pulley handle attached to your feet, exhale as you pull your knees to your chest, then inhale as you return.

Incline Leg Raise

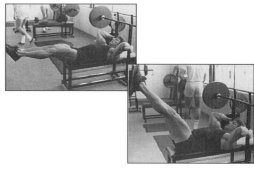

Lying back down with your legs extended off an inclined bench, exhale and slowly raise your fully extended legs to a 45-degree angle, then inhale as you lower to start.

Roman Chair Situp

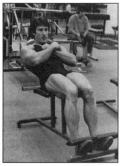 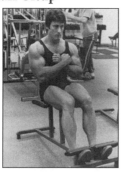

Sit on a Roman Chair with hands crossed on chest. Lean back to a 45-degree angle as you inhale slowly. Tense your abs as you exhale and lean forward until your arms touch your legs.

Incline Knee-In

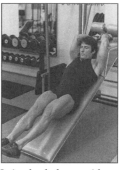 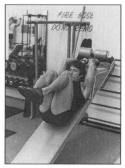

Lying back down with your legs extended off a bench, slowly exhale as you pull your knees to your chest, then inhale as you straighten your legs back out to the fully extended position.

Two-Arm Cable Crunch

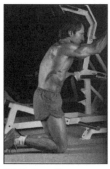 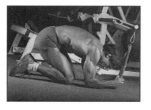

While kneeling, grasp a high pulley cable handle with both hands above your head, slowly exhale as you bend your upper body until your forearms touch the floor, then inhale as you return to the start.

AEROBICS

Stationary Bike

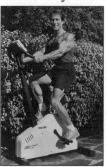

Rowing Machine

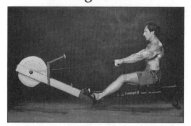

Treadmill

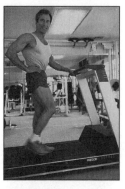

Bicycle Riding

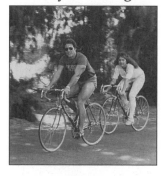

Airdyne

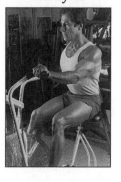

Stairclimber

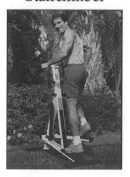

Running

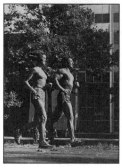

STRETCHES

Two-Arm Lat Stretch

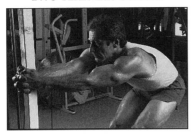

One-Arm Lat Stretch

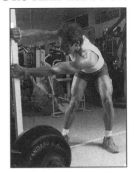

One-Leg Back Stretch

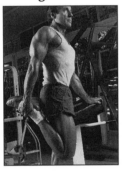

One-Leg Up Stretch

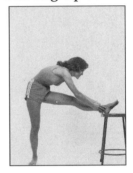

Calf Stretch

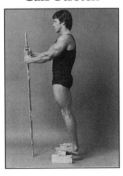

Doorway Stretch

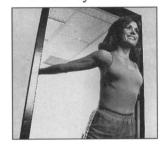

One-Arm Shoulder Stretch

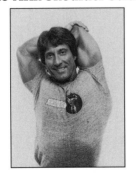

Arms Back Stretch

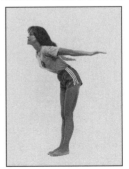

One-Arm Rear Delt Stretch

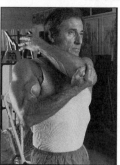

Sideways Swing

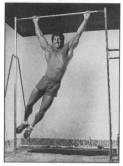

REFERENCES & RECOMMENDED READING

Akegarasu, Haya: *Shout of Buddha*
Bentov, Itzak: *Stalking the Wild Pendulum*
Bible (Moffat translation), Book of Matthew
Charters, Ann, ed.: *The Portable Kerouac*
Chinmoy, Sri: *Bird Songs*
Drub, Gendun: *Bridging the Sutras and Tantras*
Easwaran, Eknath: *The Upanishads*
Eliot, T.S. : *The Four Quartets*
Goleman, Daniel: *The Meditative Mind*
Gibran, Kahlil: *The Prophet*
Isherwood, Christopher: *How to Know God*
Jung, Carl: *Memories, Dreams and Reflections;* *The Archetypes and the Collective Unconscious*
Jung, Emma: Anima and Animus
Kerouac, Jack: Dharma Bums; On the Road; Desolation Angels, The Scripture of the Golden Eternity
Murphy, Michael: The Future of the Body
Ouspensky, P.D.: In Search of the Miraculous
Parabola Magazine: Sleep: January 1982 #1; Dreams and Seeing: 1982 #2
Remde, Harry: The House, published in A Way of Working ed. by Dooling, D.M.
Rilke, Rainer Maria: Selected Poems of Rainer Maria Rilke ed. by Robert Bly
The Selected Poetry of Rainer Maria Rilke ed. by Stephen Mitchell
Sengstan: hsin hsin ming: Verses on the Faith Mind
Shaw, Indres: World Tales
Stevens, Wallace: The Collected Poems of Wallace Stevens
The Teaching of Buddha
Thoreau, Henry David: Walden
Tonkinson, Carole, ed.: Big Sky Mind
White, John: What is Meditation?
Wilhelm, Richard: Secret of the Golden Flower
Zane, Frank: Fabulously Fit Forever Expanded

FABULOUSLY FIT FOREVER is a guide to learn the exercises described in these diaries and develop proficiency.

   This 336 page book is $13.95 + $3 postage ($4 in Canada, $10 overseas)

Frank's NEWEST audio tapes described in his diaries are the TRAIN WITH ZANE audio cassettes:

   Workout 1—Pulling muscles: Back, biceps, forearms, abs.
   Workout 2—Legs and Aerobics
   Workout 3—Pushing muscles: Chest, shoulders, triceps
   Workout 4—Get Abs

Each TRAIN WITH ZANE cassette is $14.95 or $47.85 ppd. for all four.

Also available at $14.95 each + $2 postage:
   Get Stronger
   Unwind
   Peak Performance
   Focus
   Waves of Energy
   Learn
   Sleep Sound
   Positive Attitude

Buy any three tapes, get the fourth tape FREE! $47.85 postpaid

Phone consultation is available with Frank at $50 per half hour.
   Call 760-323-7486 to schedule an appointment.

Vacation and TRAIN WITH ZANE in sunny Palm Springs
ask about private exercise, nutrition and motivational seminars with Frank.
Train with Frank and get a customized program
save years of making mistakes
learn what it takes to relax.

Visa, Mastercard, Amex, Discover orders call 800-323-7537
or send money order (faster service than check) to:
   ZANANDA INC., PO BOX 2031, PALM SPRINGS, CA 92263